PRAISE FOR *THE CAMPBELL PLAN*

"With this most worthy companion book to *The China Study*, Dr. Thomas Campbell is once again a superb guide on our journey to optimum health. What will strike the reader most is Dr. Campbell's admirable balance between confidence and humility. When he's not yet sure, he tells us why. When he is sure, he not only explains why, but also shows us how. Don't miss it."

—*Douglas J. Lisle, PhD, coauthor of* The Pleasure Trap

"*The Campbell Plan* is a terrific adjunct to *The China Study* and will ensure that your path toward better health is not only easy but truly enjoyable!"

—*Alona Pulde, MD, and Matthew Lederman, MD, authors of* The Forks Over Knives Plan *and founders of Transition to Health Center*

"*The Campbell Plan* is a clear, concise, and thorough strategy for anyone who wants to take their health to the moon following the principles of a whole-foods, plant-based diet. Who better to guide the way than Dr. Tom Campbell!!"

—*Rip Esselstyn, #1* New York Times *bestselling author of* The Engine 2 Diet *and* My Beef with Meat

"Dr. Tom Campbell expertly and creatively blends evidence-based recommendations and practical information in *The Campbell Plan*. I urge you to read this book to put the remarkable benefits of building your meals from fruits, vegetables, grains, and legumes into action. Your body (and doctor) will applaud you."

—*Amy Joy Lanou, PhD, chair and associate professor, Department of Health and Wellness, University of North Carolina, Asheville*

"The groundbreaking research of the original *China Study* helped usher in a revolution in thinking; today, the global scientific community recognizes the clear connection between healthy diets and lower risk for many cancers."

—*Marilyn Gentry, president, World Cancer Research Fund International*

"I was thrilled to read Dr. Tom Campbell's new book, *The Campbell Plan,* which transforms the scientific insights of his previous groundbreaking book, *The China Study,* into an easy-to-understand-and-apply approach to getting and staying healthy! This book will be mandatory reading for all of our patients."

—*Alan Goldhamer, DC, director, TrueNorth Health Center, Santa Monica, California*

"Reading *The Campbell Plan* puts you in the presence of a caring, experienced family physician who powerfully reveals the Standard American Diet as the chief culprit in our major disease epidemics: obesity, diabetes, high blood pressure, heart attack and stroke, and many cancers and autoimmune diseases. This is one 'doctor's appointment' you will enjoy—and benefit from all your life. Highly recommended!"

—*Michael Klaper, MD, staff physician, TrueNorth Health Center, Santa Monica, California*

"As the evidence on smoking and health became clear in the 1960s, doctors led the way by quitting smoking in record numbers. Over time it's become a standard of care to advise smokers to quit. As the evidence on a whole-food plant-based diet accumulates, more and more doctors and health-care providers will improve their diets and help their patients to do so as well. This book is a breath of fresh air."

—*Gary A. Giovino, PhD, MS, professor and chair, Department of Community Health and Health Behavior, University at Buffalo, SUNY*

"This book is a wonderful and helpful sequel to *The China Study.* Tom Campbell summarizes the research demonstrating the health benefits of a whole-food, plant-based diet (why we should change our diet) and then provides very practical advice on how to adopt such a diet, even including menu plans, recipes, and shopping lists. I highly recommend *The Campbell Plan* to health professionals, patients, and the general public."

—*Thomas L. Campbell, MD, chair, Department of Family Medicine, University of Rochester School of Medicine (no relation to the author)*

THE
CAMPBELL
PLAN

The Simple Way to Lose Weight
and Reverse Illness,
Using *The China Study's*
Whole-Food, Plant-Based Diet

THOMAS CAMPBELL, MD
CO-AUTHOR OF *THE CHINA STUDY*

FOREWORD BY T. COLIN CAMPBELL, PhD

RODALE.

For Erin, my favorite;
For Mom and Dad, the kindest revolutionaries I've ever known;
And for the patients everywhere looking to take control of their health

CONTENTS

I've presented hundreds of diet and health lectures over the last 20 to 30 years, mostly concerning the exceptional health benefits of a whole-food, plant-based (WFPB) dietary lifestyle. The world of diet and health is littered with claims and counterclaims, but a tipping point for the WFPB idea is beginning to peer above the din. Interest in this extraordinary way of achieving health is gaining unprecedented momentum. Many are wondering why they have not heard this before, while others are anxious to get started, wanting to know how best to do it. As this interest grows, questions naturally arise about the supporting evidence, in part because this idea challenges long-held, almost sacred assumptions and practices.

It is extremely important, therefore, that discussion of this evidence be articulated in a way that is, first and foremost, true to its scientific foundation. The evidence is both compelling and promising because it points a way to resolve a broad range of difficult societal problems. These problems are complex, collectively defining the human condition, both private and public. As much as any other consideration, and perhaps surprising to many, deciding what to eat goes a long way toward solving these problems. If this dietary lifestyle is done right, it means maintaining and restoring personal health, minimizing health care costs, preventing environmental degradation, limiting unnecessary violence, and reconfiguring a badly distorted food production economy. Because the root causes of these seemingly diverse problems converge on our food choices, it is paramount to ask what is the evidence for this dietary practice and how is it obtained, understood, and used?

Tom Campbell, MD, my son, is unusually prepared to tackle this question. Trained in arts and communication—theater arts was his major at Cornell University—he joined me in coauthoring *The China Study*, bringing with him skills that made our book unusually readable and, ultimately, eminently successful. That experience and the exceptionally promising evidence for this dietary lifestyle prompted him to seek a career in medicine, eventually leading to board certification in family medicine. His training in medicine, his in-depth knowledge of nutrition, and, along the way, his experience with patients in his clinic provide an unusually good combination to consider this evidence in a way that works, both for his patients and for his colleagues.

Getting the evidence right especially requires tackling the difficult issues, which generate a marketplace presence and a lot of public discussion but oftentimes with little or no supporting science. I have in mind issues like omega-3 fats (supplements versus foods?), low-carb diets (what kind of "carbs"?), gluten sensitivity (how many people need to care?), fish oil (same as whole fish? or none at all?), wheat and other cereals (good for fat bellies or a source of good fiber?), organic foods (good nutrients or bad chemicals?), and GMO foods (a promise of social good or human health risk?) among others. These are the kinds of topics that Tom clarifies using sound scientific justification.

Aside from his medical practice and his faculty association with the University of Rochester Medical School, Tom also is the executive director of our nonprofit Center for Nutrition Studies and its growing suite of online courses, offered in partnership with the nationally ranked Cornell University online program. Having coauthored *The China Study* with me and having gained a virtual graduate-level degree (three solid years) in the content and research methodology of nutritional science, Tom brings first-class nutrition information both to the public and to his physician community.

This is a book that you will want in your library. It is well written and contains a fresh and unique perspective on the more nettlesome diet and health issues. Using his writing style and analysis of the evidence, Dr. Campbell avoids a one-sided advocacy approach and instead considers various points of view. And finally the evidence is presented in a way that merges into a very readable how-to plan for making this evidence work for you, your family, your friends, your community, and the planet that we all occupy.

This way of eating and living is exceedingly important, both here and now and in the future. It *must* be made available to the public, but it must be articulated in a way that informs and is reliable. *The Campbell Plan* does just that. So please turn a page and see what I am talking about. I believe you'll like its scientific perspective, its practical advice, and its recipes. Your health and well-being stand to benefit enormously.

T. Colin Campbell, PhD

I knock on the brown door, more to announce my presence than for permission to enter. I immediately turn the door handle and push the door in to enter a fairly bright room with tan walls and a linoleum floor, the kind of floor that is sturdy and easily cleaned but lacks warmth. On my left is an exam table covered with crinkled paper, and beyond that, cupboards and a stainless steel sink where I wash my hands many times every day. To my right are two chairs and the reason I'm here: a patient, seated. I take my seat just beyond the patient on a small, swiveling stool and sign in on the computer, so I can open the patient's chart.

Even though that's when we begin talking about symptoms or concerns, I actually started my assessment the moment I walked into the room. In just a few moments I can see how alert a person is, how much weight they carry, and whether they have mobility difficulties. Did they choose the chair closer to my desk or the chair farther away? Do they stand to shake hands with stiffness and formality, or barely glance up from their cell phone until I ask two or three questions? I have no doubt they are assessing me as well. How many gray hairs do I have? Am I rushed? How do I introduce myself? And so begins the dance. I am neither unique among doctors nor particularly omniscient when it comes to reading people. It is simply what we do.

I do this as often as every 20 minutes, again and again, with people from all walks of life with all manner of complaints. But over time, I've been struck by the themes common to many of these visits.

"I want to lose weight."

"I don't want to have to take a new pill."

"I want to get rid of my pain."

"I'm tired of feeling anxious and depressed."

"I want to be healthy."

When I have these conversations and listen to people's problems, I am constantly struck by how important food choices are. Diet and emotional and mental health are deeply entwined. Poor emotional and mental health may drive poor food choices, and sometimes poor food choices actually create or exacerbate emotional and mental health problems. Obesity, diabetes, arthritic pain, heart-disease risk factors like high blood pressure or high cholesterol—all are related to diet. Yet many of my patients do not realize this when they first walk through my door. You see, I am not a diet doctor. I see normal people, most of whom do not know about my interest and background in nutrition when they first meet me. I am trained as a traditional primary care family physician. I see and treat babies, young adults, and older adults. I can do your newborn's first exam or help set up hospice orders for your dying grandparent. I do women's health. I do joint injections and skin biopsies.

Even though many of my patients—including those with diagnoses like obesity, diabetes, high blood pressure, or heart disease—do not know they should view their food choices with a critical eye, I still am invigorated by hearing about their frustrations with illness and their desire to live a better life. Don't get me wrong: It's not because I enjoy thinking about the vast number of people in our society struggling with overweight, anxiety, depression, or pain. It is because if someone is sitting in front of me expressing motivation to change their life, there is hope that I might be able to partner with and help them. There is hope that I might be able to do my job—to make a difference. Very simply, there is hope.

My patients are people like you. Why are you holding this book right now? What would you like to change? Fill in the blank: "In 1 year, with regard to my health, I would like to _____." I want you to answer these questions seriously. I'm hoping that doing so will invigorate you, because even asking and answering the questions will inspire your own hopes.

Of course, there are also plenty of barriers to success. We all know this. How many times have we started a diet and succeeded for a while, only to put the weight back on in the next few months? How many times have we joined a gym and done great for a few months, only to feel guilty as our efforts wane? How many times have we tried to eat salads every day and caved under the deprivation and hunger? For many of us, these difficulties are lifelong struggles, repeating themselves over and over without our ever getting good outcomes.

There is plenty of evidence for what makes us more likely to succeed with behavior change. At the risk of "giving away the farm" in just the first few pages of the book, I'll tell you that researchers[1] say you'll be more likely to stick with changes like those I recommend if:

1. You have clear, *personal* reasons that justify a *strong desire* to change the foods you eat.

2. You have *minimized obstacles* (environmental, cognitive, physical) to adopting a new dietary pattern.

3. You have the necessary *skills* and *confidence* to implement this new lifestyle.

4. You feel *positive* about your new eating habits and believe they will be *beneficial*.

5. Your dietary goals are consistent with your *self-image* and *social norms*.

6. You have *support* and *encouragement* from people you value and a *community* that supports your dietary changes.

I see patients fail to achieve their goals because of difficulties with each of these factors, but I believe one of the most common causes of failure is lack of knowledge. Many people would be astonished to hear that what we eat has a profound effect on our health. It is more powerful than almost anything your doctor can give you or do to you. Making the right dietary choices can turn everything to your favor. So what is the "right" dietary choice? A whole-food, plant-based diet. It is crucial to know what the optimal diet is and, therefore, what goal we're moving toward. If we don't know whether to eat low carb, vegan, or gluten free, we can make all the changes we want, but most often our efforts will be aimless and temporary: bacon and cream cheese for breakfast today, then raw salad and rice for breakfast tomorrow on the next diet. We might lose 10 pounds on one diet, then put it back on, and then lose 10 pounds with more effort on a different diet. I want you to know that there is no need to diet anymore. There is no need to yo-yo or search for the secrets. This book is about teaching you what the optimal diet is and helping you get there, without the drama.

I coauthored *The China Study,* published in 2005, with my father, the book's principal author, T. Colin Campbell, PhD. Through the lens of my dad's long, distinguished career in nutrition research, teaching, and policy making at the upper echelons of his field, our book revealed what the evidence tells us about the optimal diet. What we found was that if you want to lose weight, look better, feel better, prevent disease, regain lost health, help your heart, brain, kidneys, skin, and bowels, or lower your odds of getting cancer, then eating more fruits, vegetables, legumes, and whole grains while avoiding meats (including chicken!), dairy foods, and processed foods is the most powerful action you can take.

With the success of *The China Study*, we have seen a very large community of people change their diets and in the process radically transform their lives. I am the executive director of the T. Colin Campbell Center for Nutrition Studies, a nonprofit organization, and I have seen students who take our certificate courses at eCornell (the online course provider for Cornell University) experience aha moments—moments that forever change their lives. Once they've been given a better knowledge base, they know what is needed to be healthy and how easy and profoundly powerful it is. Physicians, dietitians, and average laypeople all have been motivated and inspired by what they've learned.

THE DISCLAIMER

Before I make too many claims, though, let me mention the disclaimer. On one of the first few pages of health books there is usually the disclaimer "This book is not intended as medical advice. Consult your personal physician before making changes in your diet or adopting any new health program."

While I have always been dismayed by the need to have disclaimers to protect our seemingly court-bound souls and wallets, the disclaimer for this particular diet book is actually more interesting than it may seem. It almost accidentally exposes the strengths of this book, and of any other book about the food you eat.

You see, the food you eat is so profoundly instrumental to your health that breakfast, lunch, and dinner are in fact exercises in medical decision making. You may have picked up this book with a singular goal, whether it's to lose weight, reduce your risk of getting heart disease, have more energy, or just feel better. But what I would like to impress upon you right away is that if you make the right food choices, you will do more to improve your health than anything else you might do. You won't just have more energy and lose weight, you also will protect your heart and lessen the risk of getting several types of cancer. You will optimize the long-term health of your brain, your kidneys, your lungs, and your gastrointestinal tract. Within days you may change how blood flows through your circulatory system and what levels of blood sugar and cholesterol that blood carries. You might even begin to reverse the course of chronic diseases that have taken years to develop. There are no panaceas that create perfect health or resolve all health problems, but choosing the right foods to eat is as close as we can get to making a single decision that will significantly improve multiple health outcomes.

Make no mistake, I do recommend that you consult a medical professional before adopting this dietary plan, especially if you are on medications; your need for those medications might change as you change your diet. Those with diabetes who follow the plan might need to reduce their dosages or eliminate the drugs entirely. Those with high blood pressure also might need to reduce how much they take, and those with high cholesterol might need to make changes, too. Readers who are already embedded in the medical system as patients might find that the course of their illness changes dramatically as they make use of the tools in this book. So, by all means, involve your doctor. Even if you consider yourself healthy, it is useful to get screening tests so you can compare your results before and after undertaking these changes.

Your dietary choices are medical choices, and therefore, changing your diet will affect you in a medical way. I'm putting this front and center: The powerful tools in this book can change your health and your life forever. So take this journey only under the counsel and with the advice of your personal physician. You've been warned.

WHO AM I?

You may be astonished by and skeptical of these grand claims that your food choices can affect all these aspects of your health. I encourage you to hold on to a healthy dose of skepticism. There are many unknowns in the science of nutrition and health, and many people who are willing to sell you just about any idea under the sun. Health product marketing is fertile ground for snake-oil salesmen, and that's as true now as it was 100 years ago.

How do you know I'm not a snake-oil salesman? I certainly could be! But I hope you'll reserve your judgment long enough to see that I'm not. My journey in nutrition started shortly after 2001, when I began writing *The China Study* with my dad. My dad grew up on a dairy farm and ended up in graduate school thinking about ways to improve high-quality animal protein production, always believing that we should consume more animal protein of an increasingly high quality. But over decades of research, he came to have a very different view. His initial scoffing at vegetarians yielded to his accepting that fruits and vegetables are healthier than anything else, and finally, later in his career, to holding the view that the healthiest diet may in fact be essentially devoid of all meat and milk.

In telling his story to the public, I became immersed in the research that linked these food choices to health. We pored over the research of other scientists and included some of their more tantalizing findings in the book. We spoke to physicians and asked what it was about our nutrition and medical systems that was obscuring the scientific findings staring us in the face. We ended up with a book with more than 700 references, many of which were reports on primary research studies that were published in medical journals.

After years of this work, I became a medical doctor. I went from thinking about nutrition and health to studying and learning about disease, diagnosis, and treatment as it is done in our current medical system. What I have found is that for all the genius and technology of our acute-care medical system, we are in fact quite poor at understanding, treating, and averting the development of chronic health problems and diseases. These problems more often than not are lifestyle related, and the current medical model addresses lifestyle issues so poorly. Our medical system essentially ignores the very powerful nutrition and lifestyle information I had just spent years learning about while my dad and I were writing *The China Study*. The reasons for this could be the subject of several books, but suffice it to say that it is not an optimal situation.

My background as a board-certified family physician and the coauthor of a very in-depth analysis of diet and health allows me to combine the best of both worlds. As a physician working within our acute-care system, I want to let individual patients know how to address their lifestyle-related chronic diseases. As I move forward in my career and see new patients, I want to offer them a set of tools to help them avoid disease, and if they already have disease, to give them the best odds of regaining their health. This book contains that set of tools.

By the end of this book, you'll know why food is so important to your health. A brief sampling of the evidence will help you understand how profound your dietary choices can be, and what foods have been shown to be the healthiest. After explaining the "why," I'll give you guidelines for knowing which foods are safe and which are toxic. You'll know not only what foods to eat, but also how to navigate the food culture that surrounds us every day, a food culture that usually sets us up for failure and sickness.

I'll offer answers to some of the most common questions I hear: Do you need to eat organic? Is fish healthy? What about gluten? And finally, I'll offer you step-by-step suggestions for grocery shopping, eating out, and cooking that will allow you to put your new knowledge into practice. All of this will lead you to the 14-day cooking and eating trial presented at the end of the book. After just a few days of reading and 14 trial days, you will possess all the necessary skills for making the most radical health improvements you likely will ever make. You will have the tools to create your best health possible.

I've cared for many patients who have lifestyle-related diseases. And though every person and situation is different, almost everyone I've met could benefit in some way from eating a healthier diet. This message is not always popular with my colleagues or my patients, but I continue to be motivated by the people I've met over the years. Patients deserve better. Patients deserve to know how to lose weight, lessen their pain, avoid taking or reduce their dosages of medications, and even reverse or slow the progression of diseases by simply choosing different breakfasts, lunches, and dinners. It is my wish that everyone could know how to be healthy. I want everyone to know how to better protect and promote their long-term health than any doctor, drug, or procedure ever could.

Throughout all of this, realize that *you are in the driver's seat*. Success is yours to grasp, and it is easier, tastier, cheaper, and more convenient than you may realize. Better health is a practice, a goal that you can achieve, and I am going to tell you how.

Part 1

FOUNDATIONS OF HEALTH

Chapter 1
The China Study

"I think you mean the high-protein diet," she said. I looked back at her, a bit confused as to why my teacher would tell me I was wrong. I probably started to disagree. "I think you mean the rats that ate more protein ran more," she said again. "But that's okay. Thank you for telling us about the experiment." She turned to the class. "Class, thank Tom for the opportunity to learn about this experiment." That was probably the first nutritional disagreement of my life, and honestly, I had no idea what was going on.

I was in grade school, standing in front of the class giving a presentation. My dad, T. Colin Campbell, PhD, had long been a nutritional biochemist who, among other things, had been conducting cutting-edge research on the influence of diet on cancer at Cornell University. He had a robust research program that was gaining national recognition, and some of his research utilized rats eating different types of diets. He had offered my teacher the opportunity to conduct a little experiment in class involving rats. Nothing pleases elementary students more than having rodents in the classroom, so of course this seemed like a perfect idea.

The experiment explored the following question: If you fed rats different levels of protein, which rats would exercise the most? Each of the rats I brought in was housed in a cage with an exercise wheel that had a counter rigged up to register the number of times the rats turned the wheel. It was like a rat pedometer. The rats would intermittently get on the wheel and run and run and run—with purpose. It made me wonder if they knew they were not going anywhere, but I suppose you could ask the same thing at your local gym. Animals just need to exercise, I guess, even if it involves not actually going anywhere.

Both groups of rats ate exactly the same dietary chow with just one variation: One group had a low-protein chow (probably about 5 percent protein) and the other group had a high-protein chow (probably about 20 percent protein). The low-protein chow had a bit more sugar to replace the protein component.

I would feed the rats faithfully and record exactly how much they exercised. My dad supplied everything, of course. As you might imagine, as an elementary school student I didn't really know what was going on. I had some very cute rats and I wrote down the wheel counter results and I fed them. It was a good life.

After a week or two, I accumulated all of my data and got my final result: The low-protein rats exercised more. I was a compulsive child, relishing the details and double-checking all my records carefully. At the end of the experiment, I stood up in front of the class and reported the data to the other sniffly kids. The rats eating the low-protein diet ran more on their wheels, I said. This was when my teacher interjected, telling me I got either the rats or the numbers mixed up, that surely I meant that the rats eating the high-protein chow exercised more. As a young student, I had no idea why my teacher would disagree with my findings. She was a wonderful teacher—very caring, enthusiastic, and nurturing. She was one of my favorite teachers.

But I certainly did not get the numbers mixed up. She hadn't recorded the exercise wheel counts; I had. How would she know what the results were? I probably told her I was actually right, but I can't remember. I was also a stubborn child. It's funny—I can't remember much about the experience of the experiment, but for some reason I have remembered the teacher telling me I got things mixed up. And so went the first nutritional disagreement of my life. I didn't know it at the time, but this was my first lesson in the absolute reverence people have for protein.

GETTING TO KNOW DAD

Despite getting to play with rats in elementary school, I was not particularly enamored with my dad's work or with nutrition early in life. As a child and adolescent, I barely knew what he did for work. I was much more interested in sports and friends. Since that time, I have traveled a long, winding path to where I am today. In my nostalgia, it is hard not to think about some of the most remarkable experiences I have had since that time, particularly during my training as a medical doctor. I will never forget the life-and-death moments I have been privy to: doing chest compressions on a man who should have been in the prime of his life; doing chest compressions on a baby born at 26 weeks of gestation not even struggling to take in the first breath. I have been the person to tell someone that their mom was dying, or their spouse was dying, or that their imaging results showed a mass likely to be cancer. I have seen jubilant tears of joy and triumph and quiet love while helping to deliver almost 100 babies. I have assisted in the operating room at a variety of surgeries on patients made sterile by the patchwork of blue drapes around the surgical field. I will never forget some of these experiences. Nor will I forget the work, the stress, or the agony of uncertainty when nothing less than perfection is expected.

These moments may seem like they have nothing to do with nutrition, but the only reason I ever lived them was because of my experience in nutrition. I did not choose at an early age to become a doctor. Instead, it was a path I chose after working with my father and being inspired to pursue a career in health. After a childhood of not being aware of what type of work my dad did and later making forays into theater and acting, even immigration law, my path dramatically changed in my midtwenties. I had the opportunity to work with my dad as coauthor of *The China Study: The Most Comprehensive Study of Nutrition Ever Conducted and the Startling Implications for Diet, Weight Loss and Long-Term Health,* in which we tell the story of his career and the most exciting results in his research. In addition, we detail the findings of many dozens of other researchers investigating diet and health. In all of this, there is a surprisingly consistent, inspiring message: Whole-food, plant-based diets are profoundly important in preventing and even treating disease.

Much of my dad's work focused on protein and cancer. Having grown up on a dairy farm and gone on to school to find out how we might produce high-quality animal protein more efficiently, he started with the same reverence for protein that my grade school teacher had. But he went on to conduct decades of experimental research on diet and cancer using a variety of experimental rodent models. The research revealed that cancer caused by a dose of a potent cancer-causing chemical can be almost entirely controlled by protein intake. In fact, one of the most provocative experiments found that early cancer growth can be turned on or off simply by changing the level of protein consumed. And guess what? High-protein diets were the most dangerous kind. The figure below shows a 12-week experiment[1] in which protein intake was changed every 3 weeks. It shows how diets composed of 5 percent protein turned off early cancer growth, whereas 20 percent protein diets promoted early cancer growth.

Perhaps the biggest surprise was that the protein that promoted cancer in these experimental models was casein, the main protein in cow's milk. Wheat[2] and soy protein in their naturally occurring forms in food do not promote cancer, even at higher levels of intake. Furthermore, protein intake affects cancer initiation and promotion in numerous ways. Dietary composition did not exert its cancer-related effects through one enzyme or one chemical; instead, it changed just about every biochemical aspect of cancer initiation and promotion that was investigated. For decades, funding sources such as the National Institutes of Health, the American Cancer Society, and the American Institute for Cancer Research awarded my dad's research team highly competitive grant money, and the results of their work were published in prestigious peer-reviewed journals.

We also wrote about one of the most comprehensive studies of diet and disease ever undertaken—the China Project, for which we named our book. A survey of 6,500 adults in 65 counties in rural China, the study, called the "Grand Prix of epidemiology" in the *New York Times,*[3] probed the relationships between 367 variables. The findings were clear: Even in

HIGH AND LOW PROTEIN INTAKE EFFECTS ON EARLY CANCER GROWTH

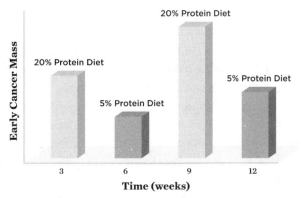

Source: Youngman LD and Campbell TC. The sustained development of preneoplastic lesions depends on high protein intake. *Nutrition and Cancer* 1992;18:131–142.

a population that consumed only small amounts of animal foods, those who consumed more animal foods had higher cholesterol levels, which in turn were linked to higher rates of diseases more common in more affluent cultures, such as several types of cancers and diabetes.[4]

In the years I spent writing and conducting library research, I learned that the argument for plant-based diets had become much more powerful than any one person's research. No single study can "prove" anything, and determining what is likely to be true requires one to survey the depth and breadth of the evidence in favor of any argument. If you're unwilling to spend a couple of years looking for the dietary advice that meets those requirements of having a broad and deep evidence base, I will tell you now that the evidence overwhelmingly supports the argument that we should be eating more unrefined plant foods and less meat, dairy, and processed foods. No other dietary recommendation even comes close in terms of comprehensive support.

Consider heart disease: We have known for more than 50 years that populations consuming more animal foods have more heart disease.[5] In fact, in many traditional plant-based cultures around the world, heart disease has historically been a very rare cause of premature death.[6, 7] However, 21st-century America is quite different. How many people with heart disease do you know? Or high blood pressure? Or high cholesterol? Of course, in modern America, heart disease and its risk factors are everywhere. But even once heart disease is advanced, we know that making a change to a healthy lifestyle alone can reverse the disease. Both Dean Ornish, MD, and Caldwell Esselstyn Jr., MD, have reversed their patients' heart disease with diet and lifestyle, and proven it with angiograms (x-rays of the heart vessels). Dr. Ornish's Lifestyle Heart Trial was a randomized, controlled trial in which he put one group of heart-disease patients in a diet and lifestyle program, without cholesterol-lowering drugs, while the other group was given standard medical care. The standard medical care group received the usual medical recommendations (medications, testing, procedures, etc.) without the intensive lifestyle program. The lifestyle group was prescribed a diet rich in fruits, vegetables, and whole grains, with almost no meat or dairy foods and no added fat, along with stress-reduction techniques, exercise, and social support. What followed was nothing less than revolutionary: Despite a lifetime of bad habits having clogged up their arteries, those in the lifestyle group began to see disease reversal within a short

CHANGES IN ARTERY BLOCKAGES WITH
DR. ORNISH'S LIFESTYLE HEART TRIAL

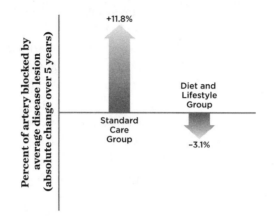

Source: Ornish D, Scherwitz LW, Billings JH, Gould L, et al. Intensive lifestyle changes for reversal of coronary heart disease. *JAMA: The Journal of the American Medical Association* 1998;280:2001–2007.

period of time. The figure above shows how the blockages in the lifestyle group shrank while the blockages in the standard care group got bigger.[8]

Diabetes is much the same story. Guess which populations have had the lowest rates of type 2 diabetes over the past 100 years? Those that eat *high*-carbohydrate, low-fat, plant-based diets.[9] And we now know that, like heart disease, we can reverse diabetes. In a study published 30 years ago, 13 of 17 diabetic participants who had required daily insulin to control their blood sugar were able to come off insulin within just 3 weeks. Of 23 patients requiring oral medication, 21 were able to discontinue their medications within 3½ weeks. When most people stop taking these blood sugar–lowering medications, their blood sugar level spikes upward. But participants in this program, even those who were stopping their medications, actually saw a decrease in their blood sugar. How did they do it? With a *high-carbohydrate*, high-fiber, low-fat diet, along with exercise[10]— the same diet plan that I present in this book.

Just take a moment and imagine that: If you are on medication for diabetes, within just 2 to 3 weeks of following the Campbell Plan, you—with your doctor's okay—might be able to get off all your diabetes medication forever! (Remember, involving your doctor prior to making your dietary change is crucial.)

Then, of course, there is the weight loss. You can eat as much as you want of the meals described in the back of this book and lose weight while you do it. Studies time and time again have found vegetarians and vegans, on average, to be thinner than their meat-eating counterparts.[11-13] In one recent large study, the researchers found that even if two people ate the same number of calories every day, a person who ate 250 more grams of meat a day would gain 4.4 pounds more every 5 years than someone getting those calories from foods other than meat.[14] Two hundred and fifty grams is perhaps the size of a steak, or a little more than a dozen chicken nuggets. The study showed that red meat, processed meats (ham, hot dogs, sausage, luncheon meats, bacon, and so on), and yes, even poultry were associated with increased weight gain.[14]

Diets containing more healthy, unrefined plants have been shown to prevent or treat a wide range of other diseases. They include kidney disease (including kidney stones), Alzheimer's dementia, gallstones, and certain cancers, including those of the breast, lung, colon, ovaries, uterus, and prostate. Listed below are some of the illnesses shown by published research[15] to be associated with improved outcomes with more plant-food intake, or worsened outcomes with more animal-food intake. If there was one pill or one surgical procedure that, without any side effects, got results like those possible with a whole-food, plant-based diet, every single person in America would want to have it.

ILLNESSES THAT MAY BE PARTLY PREVENTED OR TREATED WITH PLANT-BASED DIETS OR PLANT NUTRIENTS

High blood pressure	Obesity
High cholesterol	Alzheimer's disease
Heart disease	Parkinson's disease
Gallstones	Cataracts
Ulcers	Macular degeneration
Gastroesophageal reflux disease (GERD)	Enlarged prostate
	Oral cancer
Diabetes (both type 1 and type 2)	Lung cancer
Kidney stones	Liver cancer
Chronic kidney disease	Stomach cancer

Colorectal cancer	Chronic obstructive lung disease
Endometrial (uterine) cancer	Ulcerative colitis
Pancreatic cancer	Crohn's disease
Prostate cancer	Rheumatoid arthritis
Acne	Multiple sclerosis

Source: Campbell TM 2nd and Campbell TC. The breadth of evidence favoring a whole foods, plant-based diet: Part I: Metabolic diseases and diseases of aging. *Primary Care Reports* 2012;18:13–23.

However, in this book I won't set out the scientific argument for *why* it is so imperative to consider a whole-food, plant-based diet. I want to show you *how* to do it while answering the most common questions about the details of the diet. The process of changing your diet is tough, but it is not as hard as you might think. The new food tastes good, it doesn't cost a fortune, and it isn't hard to make. Once you settle in, you'll never look back. Part 1 of this book is an introduction to the diet and to how to think about and understand food. You'll find fundamental tips and ideas for actually making changes in your diet and lifestyle. Part 2 answers the most common questions people have about the optimal diet. Should I eat fish? What about wheat? Aren't some oils healthy? After my dad and I wrote *The China Study,* it became clear to us that some topics demand extra attention. In this section, these topics get that attention. Part 3 is the day-by-day diet plan. It gives you step-by-step instructions that are tantamount to my holding your hand through a 2-week transition that has the potential to change your life forever. By the end, you'll have the skills and knowledge you need to take control of your health.

If you get to the end and want to know more about why you should be considering a whole-food, plant-based diet, I commonly refer people back to *The China Study*. It took us 3½ years to write it. After the stressful last few months of writing, working long hours every day to be sure we would meet deadlines, I took some time to travel around the country. The day I left home, I remember having a powerful emotional response, a sense that I had come to the end of a very special project. It was special for me on several levels. By the end, I knew what my dad did throughout his career. I knew why he was so highly regarded, and why he was asked to serve on national policy committees and help shape the way Americans view food and nutrition. I knew I had been in the enviable position of spending years with a giant in the field as I learned the lessons he had gleaned during his full career. I knew how instrumental my mom had been in his work. I also knew at the time that somehow this project would shape my life for years to come.

And indeed it has. *The China Study* led my career path through medicine, through a career in which remarkable human events, both tragic and uplifting, happen routinely. Now, as a result of the experience I have in nutrition, I go beyond the traditional Western medical background and care for my patients using a more holistic approach. Once I learned what the obvious cause of our most common diseases is and learned both the art and frustration of diagnosis and treatment with pills and procedures, it has become my obligation to share the lessons I learned in writing *The China Study* with all who are interested.

While I knew that book was personally important from the moment we finished, I did not anticipate how much of a commercial success it was to become. As it turns out, people are desperately hungry for this life-changing information. Though *The China Study* is a more thoughtful book containing far more in-depth science than is included in most food-related books, it became a viral smash hit, selling more than a million copies and spreading by word of mouth to become one of the most influential diet-related books of the past 20 years. It has inspired legions of fans, including professional athletes, influential politicians, and powerful corporate leaders. I have been fortunate to have the opportunity to create meaningful improvements for individuals and society as an educator and the executive director at the T. Colin Campbell Center for Nutrition Studies, a nonprofit organization that has educated thousands of students through online programs at eCornell, Cornell University's online course provider.

BUT CAN IT BE TRUE?

At the time I'm writing this, almost nine years have passed since *The China Study* was first released. When something becomes popular and threatens what some people hold dear, there is bound to be backlash. Diet is surprisingly personal for people, and suggesting that an optimal diet might not include any meat is enough to make some people apoplectic. In the age of the Internet, there is certainly no shortage of self-proclaimed, self-taught "experts." You can find any opinion you would like to believe on the Internet. Unfortunately, it can be less apparent what people's motivations are. Who is providing funding to whom, and who is really generating the information you read online? There are enormous financial interests involved in the food industry. In fact, the food industry is arguably the most powerful industry on the planet. After all, just about the only thing every American must purchase and consume every day is food. Unfortunately, the biggest food conglomerates by far are animal-agriculture and processed-food businesses.

All this is to say that there have been many distractions and sources of confusion along the way to our success. A great deal of the confusion over diet and health can be attributed to the making of a fundamental mistake: looking at details out of context. For example, when we were writing *The China Study*, we visited with a well-respected researcher who was doing work on conjugated linoleic acid, or CLA. CLA is a fatty acid present in beef and dairy foods that has shown some evidence of inhibiting cancer formation. This research generated endless headlines proclaiming that beef and dairy foods might inhibit cancer formation. When we visited with this researcher—one who for much of his career had been a friend to the animal-food industry—he admitted, with an almost ironic humor, that any health effects attributed to CLA would only be relevant in a pharmaceutical way. In other words, he knew that in the small amounts that CLA was present in foods, it did not have a relevant health effect. It could be protective only if people isolated the chemical and ingested large amounts of it (which has been done, of course). And yet the media continued to drive sales of lots of beef and dairy foods by trumpeting the out-of-context findings of research on CLA, and the scientist continued providing the research fodder backing it.

In the same way, the small crowd of people who have pushed back most vigorously against *The China Study* (virtually none of whom are clinicians or scientists) use details out of context to try to derail the message. For example, if some correlations in the China Project (the actual scientific study) do not align with the researchers' general findings, detractors make the case that the whole study is flawed, and therefore that all of the research that T. Colin Campbell has done is flawed, and therefore the whole argument presented in *The China Study* is flawed. Can you see the logic in that? I cannot. Let us assume that the China Project does not prove anything (which is, ironically, an idea that the researchers would all agree with). That leaves still hundreds of other studies, from hundreds of other researchers, that lend their weight to the breadth and depth of evidence in support of more plant-based diets. Any Internet detractors of *The China Study* tend to ignore this breadth and depth of research. They would have to go through hundreds of papers and find flaws in order to disagree with hundreds of different scientists in an effort to negate mountains of evidence, all from their home computer without training in science or medicine. If one can write a few catchy blogs, one can try to discredit one person, but to take down the depth and breadth of evidence in favor of eating more plants—you won't see that anywhere, even on the Internet.

In fact, in the past 9 years the evidence in support of a whole-food, plant-based diet has only become deeper and broader. Another randomized, controlled trial showed yet again that diabetes can be successfully treated.[16] In addition, there has been promising research on the treatment of prostate cancer with diet and lifestyle. Men with low-grade prostate cancer can actually lower their levels of PSA (prostate-specific antigen, the blood biomarker used to follow prostate cancer progression) with diet and lifestyle alone.[17] This same research demonstrated that a whole-food, plant-based diet might control genetic expression, turning off the bad cancer genes and turning on the good genes to treat prostate cancer.[18] The caps at the ends of our chromosomes (called telomeres), which protect the genes on the chromosomes, degrade over time as we age and experience stress and disease. Perhaps the most remarkable finding of recent research is that, when compared to a normal American diet, a whole-food, plant-based diet in combination with other lifestyle changes can actually reverse this degrading process.[19]

Another hot topic is the enormously complex microbial system residing in our intestines. We are learning that these bacteria likely play a major role in our health and disease. Evidence from animal studies now shows that diet plays the primary role in determining whether we have a good bacteria profile or bad bacteria profile.[20, 21] Low-fat, fiber-rich, plant-based diets are linked to healthier bacterial communities.[22, 23] Most impressively, evidence shows that after just 1 day of eating bad food, the kinds of bacteria in the intestines will change dramatically.[23] In a separate series of headline-making studies, researchers found that gut bacteria play a key role in turning a nutrient in red meat, L-carnitine, into a heart-disease promoter referred to as TMAO.[24] It is yet another way that chronic animal-food consumption promotes heart disease. Vegans and vegetarians participating in the study didn't have the gut bacteria necessary to create the nasty changes.[24]

GRADE SCHOOL AND ONWARD

I went from a childhood of eating sausage and meat loaf to an adolescence of being the somewhat strange semivegetarian kid. I knew food was important, but I never really cared. I just ate what was fed to me. As an adult, I learned about the science that shows that in many of our most pressing personal and societal problems, food is a central issue. As a doctor, it is now my obligation to share that information. When I think back to my elementary school teacher, I have to chuckle at my first lesson in nutrition. I had no idea what I was stepping in when I suggested that rats fed a lower-protein diet had more energy; now I know. Rather than being confused by her assumption, I might now suggest to her that rats or humans eating lesser amounts of animal protein and more plant-based foods might have not only more energy, but also lower odds of developing obesity, diabetes, high blood pressure, heart disease, kidney disease, liver disease, brain disease, and prostate, breast, and colon cancers. Their genes are going to "look" younger; even their poop and the bacteria in their poop are more aligned with good health. Humans are not all that different from rats in many ways. And while I do not go about my day thinking about my odds of developing disease or the quality of my poop, I do like the idea of being able to run on that exercise wheel a few more times every day. That means more energy, more vitality, more fun, more success, and more health.

Chapter 2

Cavemen Counting Carbs

Where does an 800-pound gorilla sit? Anywhere it wants to, of course. Gorillas are among the more powerful plant eaters in the world. Like other primates, they get the vast majority of their energy from plants: green leaves, stems, fruits, and vines. In reality, there are no 800-pound gorillas; males grow to about 300 to 400 pounds, and females are significantly smaller. They are among our closest genetic relatives in the Animal Kingdom, along with chimpanzees and bonobos.

In the United States, of course, we will only ever see them in zoos. Unfortunately, most zoo gorillas are not in ideal health. Mysteriously, they are getting sick and dying from heart disease. Their heart disease is not the result of the same process that occurs in human heart disease, however.[1] Instead, a gorilla's heart muscle becomes fibrotic, which means the muscle becomes more leathery and less responsive, coordinated, and elastic. When this happens, the gorilla's heart can't pump blood as well and the gorilla may go into heart failure or have a problem where the electrical messages that tell the heart to pump get crossed and the heart doesn't beat properly, causing an arrhythmia that can be fatal. No one really knows why this epidemic of heart disease is plaguing gorillas in US zoos, but thoughts have turned to dietary causes.

Zoos in the United States traditionally feed gorillas a varied diet of mostly plants, including fruits and vegetables, along with commercially prepared processed biscuits and small amounts of foods from animal sources.[2] Unfortunately, this is unlike their natural diet. The zoo diets, and the biscuits and animal foods in particular, are much lower in fiber and higher in fat compared to gorillas' natural diet in the wild.[2-4] In the wild, gorillas eat massive amounts of fiber, which is fermented in the colon to make short-chain fatty acids, which in turn actually provide significant caloric energy to the gorilla.[4]

Could gorilla heart disease result from the unnatural diet in zoos? We know, for example, that captive gorillas have significantly higher cholesterol than wild gorillas.[5] In one of the more intriguing recent experiments,[3] scientists fed gorillas diets of much more plant matter while avoiding biscuits. The natural diets had much more volume, more fiber, and less processed starch and sugar. As a consequence, the gorillas spent more time feeding throughout the day and their health appeared to improve. Their cholesterol and insulin levels decreased and their weight decreased by 40 to 70 pounds, approaching a weight more consistent with that typical for wild gorillas.[3]

The million-dollar question is whether this will impact chronic diseases, including heart disease, in zoo gorillas. At this point it's too early to tell, but these findings certainly are hopeful.

FROM GORILLAS TO CAVEMEN

Unfortunately, some humans have weighed well over 800 pounds, though it is obviously not a reflection of their power or strength. It is a reflection of the epidemic of obesity in our society, a reflection of how easy it is to acquire calories with output of almost no energy. In addition to widespread obesity, we have rampant cardiovascular disease. This is our number one killer. Can we approach these epidemics with the same thinking that scientists applied to the health of zoo gorillas? Can we simply try to find our "natural" diet, the diet that sustained us in the wild, and then adopt that diet in the hopes that we can cure these chronic disease scourges?

This rationale is everywhere. It is part of the premise behind several diet trends, including diets described as high protein, Paleo, "primal," and even wheat free. This argument indirectly informs the discussion about grass-fed meat as well as the "locavore," farm-to-table movement. Each of these different diet trends comes at this argument from a different angle, but I frequently see repeated the idea that any particular trend is right because that is what our Paleolithic ancestors did.

The premise is that if we could simply return to the natural Stone Age diet we evolved on from about 2.5 million years ago to 10,000 years ago, we would return to Stone Age health. Based on modern hunter–gatherer societies and their lack of common Western chronic diseases such as obesity, diabetes, and premature cardiac death, cavemen are proposed to have been free of these same chronic diseases.[6] In reality, Stone Age health is a bit of an oxymoron. Throughout the Paleolithic period, humans were lucky to live past 30 years of age,[7] and even at the end of the Paleolithic period, within the past 50,000 years, humans rarely lived past 40.[8] This short life span had nothing to do with chronic disease, of course, and everything to do with infections, trauma, and the increased danger of everyday life. As soon as something happened that limited your mobility, for example, you likely were a goner. As Erik Trinkaus theorizes in the *Proceedings of the National Academy of Sciences,* "Under these conditions, it is likely that older individuals [as in 30-somethings] with reduced mobility were left behind, to die and have their remains consumed by the ubiquitous carnivores on the landscape."[8]

Cheery times, indeed!

Let's assume that cavemen were indeed free of even the early signs of chronic disease (prior to twisting an ankle and being consumed by the ubiquitous carnivores). This is an unknown assumption, but they certainly seem likely to have been slim, strong, and without any signs of diabetes or symptomatic heart disease. What was their diet? Loren Cordain, PhD, a widely published researcher in this area and author of *The Paleo Diet,* suggests that a little more than half of their calories came from animal foods—all parts of lean, wild animals, including fish.[9] The rest of the diet was food you might walk out into the bushes and gather: fruits, vegetables, nuts, seeds, etc. This argument is derived from data on subsistence economies from a large number of hunter–gatherer societies studied over the past 100 years or so, which have been assembled in a publication called the *Ethnographic Atlas.*[9, 10] Dr. Cordain notes that fatty domesticated meats, dairy foods, all grains, salty foods, sugars (except for a little honey), and all legumes were not part of the diet, and therefore should be avoided.[11] (Oddly, though added oils were clearly not part of cavemen diets, olive oil is a common ingredient in most modern-day "Paleo" recipes.[11]) If we do this, we too can be lean, strong, and free of metabolic disease, so goes the argument.

I actually very much like certain aspects of this diet and this argument for achieving optimal health. It has a strongly intuitive appeal. I find it to be better supported scientifically than many of the popular diet beliefs in our culture. Unfortunately, though, I see major flaws in the argument that remain unresolved, and this stops me from recommending any of the most popular diets touting Paleolithic principles. I actually continue to fear that these high-protein, whole grain–phobic diets are downright dangerous.

THE POSITIVE

The high-protein Paleo diets, followed properly, are a dramatic departure from the typical American diet. In essence, a Paleo diet requires you to eat *real* food, as provided by Mother Nature. The vast majority of Americans eat artificial food, more similar to factory concoctions than a plant or animal that might be found in the wild. The table on page 18 is an unfortunate list of the top 20 most-consumed food groups and what percentage of the total energy consumed by an average American comes from that group.[12]

Of the top 20 foods consumed in the United States, only the lean meats, nuts, and seeds are allowable on a true Paleo-based diet. That means that almost all of the top 20 foods that we usually eat, from the sweet desserts to the white flour breads and rolls to the sugary sodas and beyond go straight into the garbage can. No more cookies! This is a phenomenally healthy thing, as these ultrarefined foods are devoid of any redeeming nutritional qualities, which you'll see in the next chapter. So now that we've eliminated the majority of the diet in America, what do you replace it with? Largely, you replace this junk with non-starchy fruits and vegetables. That's right, a Paleo diet that's true to the published theory includes large amounts of fruits and vegetables.

What happens if the average American takes all the processed junk food out of their diet and largely replaces it with plates of non-starchy, vitamin-rich fruits and vegetables? Their intake of fiber should go through the roof and their intake of many minerals and vitamins should go through the roof. Perhaps, then, it is unsurprising to see that there are studies showing short-term benefits to a Paleo-based diet, including results showing at least weak benefits for weight loss, blood pressure, and blood sugar control.[13–16]

THE TOP 20 FOOD GROUP CONTRIBUTORS TO AMERICANS' OVERALL ENERGY INTAKE

FOOD GROUP	% OF TOTAL ENERGY CONSUMED
Grain-based desserts	6.4
Yeast breads	6.0
Chicken and chicken mixed dishes	5.6
Soda/energy/sports drinks	5.3
Pizza	4.6
Alcoholic beverages	3.8
Pasta and pasta dishes	3.8
Mexican mixed dishes	3.7
Beef and beef mixed dishes	3.0
Dairy desserts	2.9
Potato/corn/other chips	2.6
Burgers	2.5
Reduced-fat milk	2.4
Regular cheese	2.3
Ready-to-eat cereals	2.3
Sausage, franks, bacon, and ribs	2.3
Fried white potatoes	2.2
Candy	2.2
Nuts/seeds and nut/seed mixed dishes	2.0
Eggs and egg mixed dishes	1.8

Source: National Cancer Institute. Mean intake of energy and percentage contribution of various foods among US population, by age, NHANES 2005–06. October 18, 2013. http://appliedresearch.cancer.gov/diet/foodsources/energy/table1a.html.

THE NEGATIVE

And yet, I'm not a Stone Age advocate. Why not? My first major concern is that we don't know for sure what they were eating 500,000 years ago. We can make conjectures based on relatively recent hunter–gatherers, but there's an awful lot of guesswork with this approach. The dietary data for hunter–gatherers is based on societies that largely had vanished by the mid-1900s. It was collected by a wide variety of ethnographers—most of them untrained in nutrition—in nonstandardized ways.[17] Even though Dr. Cordain has suggested that the "natural" diet is up to 65 percent animal foods, S. Boyd Eaton, MD, the father of the Paleo trend, suggested 15 years earlier that there is evidence to suggest that perhaps 35 percent of the typical hunter–gatherer diet was animal foods.[18]

Beyond trying to assess recent hunter–gatherer diets from records kept by non-nutritionists 100 years ago, we can also assess the Paleo diet with standard archeological methods. But this is imperfect as well. Stone hunting tools and bones can be preserved throughout history, but plant remains? Of course these are not preserved.[17, 19] Chemical isotope analyses of human bones have also been used as a way to understand how high on the food chain humans were, but this has also generated controversy because the results can be affected by more than just food intake.[20–22]

Perhaps most interestingly, recent evidence shows that people actually ate grass seeds and legumes and starch-rich plant parts for many tens of thousands of years prior to the agricultural revolution,[23, 24] even almost 100,000 years prior to the development of agriculture.[25] These are big no-nos on the modern Paleo diets, but this evidence suggests that these foods have been part of our evolution for much longer than originally thought. Recently, other types of chemical analysis have suggested that about 3 million years ago there was a shift to consuming energy derived from grasses.[26] Whether these ancient ancestors ate the grasses themselves or ate grass-consuming animals is unknown.[26]

Another thing that bothers me is that there is little discussion about being in an environment of scarcity in the Paleolithic period. Did Paleolithic people experience intermittent starvation, fasting, and inadequate calorie intake, particularly in the context of enormous daily physical exertion? This certainly seems possible. How does this impact our interpretation of the healthfulness of the Paleo diet? We've known for a long time that forced calorie restriction leads to protection against cancer in animal models, for example.[27] Is it possible that the theorized protection from chronic disease during Paleolithic times is more related to significant intermittent calorie restriction than to the actual dietary components themselves? Is it possible that what we really are learning from ancient diets is simply that if you are sometimes on the edge of starvation, any calorie is a good calorie, and that intermittent food scarcity will prevent early-onset chronic disease? Strangely, this line of questioning is absent from many modern-day Paleo prescriptions. Instead, I see the recommendation that we should eat meat at every single meal and frequently consume added oils, even in our modern environment of physical inactivity and calorie overabundance.

In our investigation of exactly what the Paleo diet and lifestyle were, let's agree on some basics: There was no *one* Paleo diet, a fact that everyone readily accepts. Peoples' diets varied dramatically based on region, climate, season, and ecological community. While some people ate mostly animals, others ate mostly plants. No human species evolved in the past couple of million years on a strictly vegetarian, or vegan, diet, but we are descended from species that millions of years ago likely consumed diets absolutely dominated by plants,[28] similar to most primates today. Humans can get nourishment from a wide variety of plants and animals, with amazing adaptability. I think most of us can agree on these facts.

But here's my big question: Who cares? The hypothesis that we need to find our natural diet is interesting, but when the rubber hits the road, the biggest problem with the Paleo diet is that modern nutritional research conducted over the past 100 years on modern humans has been consistently in favor of consuming more plants and less animals. Populations consuming the most carbohydrates historically have had lower rates of diabetes.[29] Vegans and vegetarians are slimmer[30] in observational studies, and one study has shown that the more meat people eat, even with the same calorie intake, the more weight people gain.[31] Strict vegetarian diets have been shown to reverse advanced heart disease,[32, 33] diabetes,[34, 35] and prostate cancer.[36, 37] Paleo-prohibited legumes have been shown to substantially improve blood sugar control in diabetic patients,[38] and intake of Paleo-prohibited whole grains has been linked to reduced rates of diabetes, obesity, cardiovascular disease, and certain types of cancer.[39, 40] High-carbohydrate, high-grain diets have been shown to rapidly and dramatically reverse diabetes.[41] In animal models, increasing amounts of animal protein have been shown to promote cancer,[42] kidney failure,[43-45] and gallstones.[46] A low-carbohydrate, high-protein diet in mice has been shown to promote atherosclerosis (heart disease)[47] even when blood cholesterol levels don't change significantly. Gut bacteria have been found to produce a heart-disease-promoting chemical, TMAO, from a nutrient in red meat, L-carnitine.[48] A review study found that the more meat people eat, the *higher* their risk of diabetes.[49] And lastly, low-carbohydrate and high-protein dietary patterns in two different human populations have been linked to an increased risk of death.[50, 51]

Are you starting to get the picture? These are just a *tiny fraction* of the studies that support eating more plants, including whole grains and legumes, and less animals. So when high-protein Paleo advocates suggest eating 35 percent of your calories as protein, most of which is from meat, at every meal when the recommended amount has always been about 10 percent of calories, I get very nervous. When these same advocates suggest avoiding all starchy plants, like whole grains, beans, and tubers, which have been dietary staples for the healthiest, longest-lived populations around the world, I get very nervous. By following a Paleo-based diet you are putting your life at the mercy of a hypothesis still full of uncertainties. The diet may have some short-term benefits, particularly compared to the standard American fare. It may yet shape our understanding of the optimal diet in important ways. But at this time, these Paleo-based diets fly in the face of evidence gathered by modern-day nutritional science about the healthiest lifelong dietary patterns. This makes me very nervous, and it should you, too.

FROM CAVEMAN TO CARBOHYDRATES

One popular idea that overlaps frequently with a Paleo-inspired argument is the low-carbohydrate diet trend. As far as trends go, low carb has been pervasive and persistent. There is a long history of carbohydrate-restricted diets in American medicine and weight loss. When we wrote *The China Study,* the Atkins Diet was just coming to the end of its wild popularity. Other diets, like the South Beach Diet and the Dukan Diet, came to replace it, putting a fresh, sexy face on the same old worn-out trend. Both the Paleo-type diets and the low-carb diets are high-protein plans, with the protein being supplied almost entirely by animal foods. But the low-carb diets have no restrictions on fatty foods or dairy foods and do not include as many fruits and vegetables as Paleo diets, as they aim for more-extreme restriction of carbohydrates.

Mountains of scientific evidence have been totally ignored in the writing of these books. In one of the most popular carb-hating books of the past decade, the author writes, "My concern was not with my patients' appearance: I wanted to find a diet that would help prevent or reverse the myriad of heart and vascular problems that stem from obesity. I never found such a diet. Instead, I developed one myself."[52] The very clear, unfortunate implication is that there is no research supporting a heart-disease-reversal diet. But by the time this popular book had been written there had been articles[32, 33, 53, 54] published in the *American Journal of Cardiology,* the *Journal of Family Practice, The Lancet,* and *JAMA: The Journal of the American Medical Association,* all of which detailed dietary reversal of even advanced heart disease as judged by radiologists reading angiograms. In other words, the results weren't based just on cholesterol results or any other blood test, they were based on radiologists looking at the sizes of blockages in the heart arteries and finding that the blockages were shrinking in the dietary treatment participants. The diets that did this, of course, were almost exclusively plant-based diets, with little or no dairy and no meat whatsoever and no added fat. They were the diets of Dr. Dean Ornish and Dr. Caldwell Esselstyn. They were very-high-carbohydrate diets.

But despite the numerous misleading statements these books contain and their authors' ignoring of mountains of research, there is a real body of research supporting low-carb diets for some outcomes. Low-carbohydrate diets can have beneficial short-term effects on some of the risk factors for metabolic disease, such as obesity and levels of certain types of cholesterol.[55] In other words, you might lose weight, lower your blood sugar, and improve your cholesterol profile on a low-carbohydrate diet in the short term. Note, however, that I've had a patient achieve some of those same short-term benefits by getting toxic doses of radiation during cancer therapy. But unfortunately, low-carb diets have never been shown to have long-term benefits. They've never been shown to reverse plaque buildup in coronary arteries, despite the dramatic claims made in some of the popular books.

In fact, I have serious concerns about the long-term health of the cardiovascular systems of those people who adopt low-carbohydrate diets. I mentioned a few studies a few pages back that are worth elaborating on here. In 2009 a study evaluating different diets in mice was published.[47, 56] There were three groups of mice, each of which was fed a different diet. One group got standard chow (high carbohydrate, lower fat), another got a "Western diet" chow (high fat, higher cholesterol), and yet a third got a low-carbohydrate diet (low carbohydrate, high protein, and the same fat and cholesterol as the Western diet). The mice eating a low-carbohydrate diet had significantly less weight gain than either of the other groups. Blood cholesterol was not significantly different between the mice eating the Western diet and those on the low-carbohydrate diet, but low-carb mice had lower blood glucose levels. If we stopped this discussion there, we could sell a diet book to the mouse masses promising weight loss, lower blood sugar, and (presumably) less diabetes. Is this sounding familiar? But let us not stop there.

After 12 weeks, the mice were killed and researchers took a look at their aortas (the major blood vessel from the heart to the rest of the body).

They found, remarkably, that the low-carb mice had about *twice* the amount of arterial plaque as the Western-diet mice. To say it another way, they had about 200 percent of the gunky blood vessel plaque that the Western-diet mice had! Both groups had much more heart disease than the standard-chow mice. How was this possible? The measurements of the intermediate risk factors had seemed so safe and promising in the low-carb group compared to those in the Western-diet group.

One of the things the researchers measured in these mice was something called endothelial progenitor cells (EPCs). Without getting bogged down in details, EPCs are made in your bone marrow and they repair and bolster the endothelial cells that line your blood vessels. This is a pretty important task, as you might guess. The mice on the low-carb diets had a dramatic reduction in EPCs circulating in their blood. Researchers also looked in the bone marrow and found the same thing: Low-carb mice weren't making the cells required to repair and reinforce their blood vessels. In addition, the low-carb mice were found to have less ability to form new blood vessels when their blood flow was challenged.

Make no mistake: The low-carb diet was destroying the cardiovascular systems of these mice, though they were thinner and had unchanged or improved levels of cholesterol, glucose, and insulin.

Perhaps it should come as no surprise that humans at risk for metabolic disease who eat more of a low-carbohydrate dietary pattern have more-poorly functioning small arteries.[57] How about the fact that in a study[58] of 40,000 people who were followed for 20 years, those who ate the fewest carbohydrates had the highest risk of getting diabetes? In a study group of 1,000 older men in Sweden, those eating the least carbohydrate content and the most protein had a higher risk of death and, in particular, an even higher risk of death from cardiovascular disease.[59] Another large study[60] found a higher risk of death among people eating in a low-carb-diet pattern if they were replacing carbohydrates with animal foods. A study[50] of Swedish women found lower carbohydrate intake and higher protein intake predicted a higher rate of death, particularly cardiovascular death. And a study[51] in Greece found the same thing: low-carb-and-high-protein dietary patterns are linked to an increased risk of death, including from cardiovascular causes and cancer.

Enough already! Do you get the picture? You can do a low-carb diet for weight loss in the short term and it may very well work. You can also do cocaine, amphetamines, chemotherapy, or toxic radiation exposure to lose weight. But I'm very concerned, based on lots of evidence, that you'll be increasing your risk of death. I also have doubts that it will lead to long-term weight loss. I have met many patients who lost weight on low-carb diets and lamented that they then put it all back on. I haven't even scratched the surface of the more than 100 years of evidence showing the dangers of high protein consumption for your kidneys. Similarly, I haven't even scratched the surface regarding the mountain of evidence showing the benefits of the diet opposite to a low-carb diet: a diet of whole plant foods, very high in carbohydrates and low in fat.

There is a kernel of truth in most of the successful dietary messages in popular culture, and low-carbohydrate messages are no exception. As I pointed out earlier, we eat vast quantities of nutritionally deficient, highly refined carbohydrates, including lots of sugar and lots of refined flours. Avoiding these is a good thing and will improve your health. But exchanging the junky carbs for bacon or eggs in rotation every other day along with snacks of ham-and-turkey roll-ups and dairy in abundance may lead to your demise.

One final point: Many popular diet book authors sell their own expensive, complex blends of branded supplements to go along with their diets, a practice with even less scientific justification than their dietary recommendations. This is a major red flag for me, and it should be for you, as well. The commercial success of some of these low-carb diet books hawking supplements exposes one truism in our culture: We love to hear good things about our bad habits. Indeed it is extremely profitable to promote bad habits in the name of health. Unfortunately, that doesn't make the bad habits any less bad.

Don't count calories, don't hate carbs, don't go to the Stone Age. Simply eat real food, healthy food, and find ways to love every bit of food and the health that results. It will become a lifelong habit and you can leave the yo-yoing behind.

Chapter 3

The Three Food Groups

R emember the four food groups? I remember learning something about these as a little kid and even then, having no concept of calories or vitamins or minerals, I understood the recommendations right away. They were so simple. You could look at the poster and pretty much instantly assess whether your meal was adequate. Are you eating some meat, dairy, fruit or veggie, and bread or grain? A steak, rice pilaf, a glass of milk, and green beans was a perfect meal and it was immediately obvious. While the nutritional recommendations of more recent government schemes (pyramids, plates, etc.) have improved, I'm not sure anything has ever been as accessible as the basic four food groups.

I would like to make your understanding of nutrition even more accessible, if that's possible. I want to introduce you to the three food groups. They are:

1. Animal products

2. Processed plant fragments

3. Whole plants

You should be able to categorize most things in the grocery store into one of these food groups by asking two questions:

1. Is this product from a plant or an animal?

2. If it is a plant, is this similar to what I could find on a tree or bush or in the dirt on a farm?

Some obvious examples:

Mozzarella cheese: It's processed from the milk of a cow, so it's an animal product.

Doughnut: It's not an animal, and it doesn't resemble any plant you might find in the dirt, so it's likely a collection of processed plant fragments.

Asparagus: In the produce section it is a whole plant. It might as well have been harvested just prior to appearing on the shelf.

The animal group and the whole-plant group are easy. But it gets a bit trickier in the processed plant fragment group. What do I mean by "processed"? Being processed means that mechanical or chemical steps were taken to isolate certain components of the original plant. For example, you can start with a whole sugar beet pulled from the ground and ship it off to a processing plant. It is sliced up and the pieces are put into a diffuser machine where water helps to separate the sugar from the fibrous material, or pulp, of the beet. The pulp is sent away to become animal feed. The raw juice is combined with certain chemicals to remove impurities and then gasses may be bubbled through the juice to remove more impurities. Then the liquid goes through further processes of boiling and drying and crystallization to end up as the final product: sugar. Through this processing of the beet, almost all the components and ingredients of the original plant are stripped away until we just have sugar: a single fragment of the original plant. The doughnut in our example above has sugar, oil, white flour, and possibly other ingredients, each of which is simply an isolated fragment of the original plant.

There are different degrees of processing, which makes this a little tricky. Oils and sugar represent the ultimate processing results. Those mostly are just single components derived from a whole plant. But there are things like brown rice pasta in the health-food section of your store. The pasta is made of whole brown rice, perhaps with some rice bran added, perhaps some other more minor ingredients. These ingredients, which are mostly whole plants, are ground up to resemble pasta shapes and to cook like pasta. Is this refined? It has been mechanically reshaped, but if you read the label, the major ingredients of the food are whole plants, so I would consider the product to be almost equivalent to a whole plant.

Another area of confusion is ready-made meals. In these you'll likely find combinations of all three food groups. For example, a frozen pizza has lots of refined white flour (processed plant fragment), a lot of cheese (animal product), and the toppings, which might be meat (animal product) and/or vegetables (whole plants). There also is tomato sauce, which is likely a relatively unprocessed form of tomatoes (whole plant), and oil (processed plant fragment), salt, and spices. In terms of the energy in this food, as with most of the traditional frozen-food meals, the calories mostly come from processed plant fragments (white flour, oils) and animal products (cheese, meat toppings) with a very small contribution from whole, unprocessed plants (tomato sauce and possible vegetable toppings).

Thinking of food in terms of these basic three food groups takes a bit of practice. Once you can think about food in this way, however, it becomes very easy to understand what foods you should eat and what foods you should stay away from. The foods that have been shown to offer benefits for almost every organ system in your body are whole plants: fruits, vegetables, whole grains and starches, and legumes. The foods to avoid? The animal foods and the refined plant fragments.

NUTRIENT DIFFERENCES

I think the clearest way to illustrate the differences among these food groups is to look at their nutrient content. Traditionally we describe the health value of a food by naming and quantifying the food's nutrients. Why do we hear that milk is healthy? Because it contains calcium and protein. Why do we hear that beans are healthy? Because they contain fiber and protein. It is an overly simplistic way to think about food, but much of the body of nutritional research has been done on individual nutrients and it can provide a useful framework for assessing a food. So let's compare the three food groups in terms of nutrients. The table on page 28 shows the nutrient content of 500 calories' worth of a sample of whole plants compared to the nutrients in 500 calories of animal products and 500 calories of processed plant fragments, or refined plants. As you can easily see, there are enormous differences.

Macronutrients (Protein, Lipid, Carbohydrate)

You can think of the macronutrients as the major "bulky" nutrients that provide the energy of food. We've all heard of them: protein, fat, and carbohydrates. Let's start with protein. Based on many decades of research and recommendations, getting at least 12.5 grams of protein from every 500 calories will be more than enough to meet all your needs. If you look at the table, you'll see the whole-plant sample has 29 grams of protein, *more than double* the recommended minimum amount. So the first important lesson from this study of nutrient comparisons is that *most whole plants are high-protein foods*.

NUTRIENT CONTENTS OF SAMPLES
FROM THE THREE FOOD GROUPS

	WHOLE PLANTS	ANIMAL FOODS	REFINED PLANTS
Protein (g)	29	51	6.5
Lipid (g)	6	34	21
Carbohydrate (g)	97	8.6	72
Fiber (g)	27	0	1.8
Calcium (mg)	410	250	31
Iron (mg)	8.4	3.5	0.9
Potassium (mg)	2,600	1,200	350
Vitamin C (mg)	440	0	4.3
Folate (mcg)	640	64	15
Vitamin B$_{12}$ (mcg)	0	5.2	0
Vitamin A (IU)	25,000	680	18
Cholesterol (mg)	0	410	0

Whole plant blend: *100 calories each of mango, pea, broccoli, kale, oats*
Animal food blend: *100 calories each of whole milk, chicken, beef, salmon, egg*
Unenriched refined plant blend: *100 calories each of potato chips, spaghetti, cola, doughnut, Italian dressing*

Source: Calculated from the USDA National Nutrient Database for Standard Reference Release 27

In fact, gorillas in the wild, who get essentially all of their calories from plants, namely fruits and leaves, get 30 percent of their calories from protein during times of the year when they consume a high-leaf diet due to low fruit availability.[1] A whole-plant-based diet can actually be high in protein.

Animal foods contain even more protein in smaller packages. Conversely, processed plant fragments are deficient in protein. In creating refined sugar and refined oil products, food makers have mechanically and chemically removed the parts of the original plants containing protein. Refined grains, including different types of flour, do retain protein, but most other refined plant products are severely protein deficient.

Fat (various types of lipids) is present in whole plants, but to a much lesser degree than in either refined plants or animal foods. A whole-plant diet with no added fat gets about 10 percent of its calories from fat. There is natural fat in those veggies, beans, and grains—just not that much. This corrects another common misperception that a whole-food, plant-based diet is fat free; it is not.

Animal foods, on the other hand, are naturally high in fat. In the sample shown in the table above, about 60 percent of the calories come from fat. For people who only eat whole plants and animals (a Paleo diet, for example), the amount of fat they eat is generally a representation of how many animal foods they eat, unless they eat lots and lots of nuts or coconuts or another high-fat plant.

Processed plant foods often have pure fat (oil) added to the ingredients. In the sample shown in the table opposite, about 40 percent of the calories in the processed plant fragment foods come from fat.

And lastly, carbohydrates, vilified by the high-protein-diet gurus, are abundant in plant foods. In fact, whole plants have the most carbohydrate. Carbohydrates are vital sources of energy and, when consumed in nutrient-rich whole plants with lots of fiber, will give you excellent health. Despite the negative picture we have of eating "carbs" in the United States, it has been shown many times over many years that the populations around the world with the lowest rates of the various diseases of affluence (obesity, certain cancers, cardiovascular diseases, etc.) consume the highest-carbohydrate diets. Carbohydrates that come from processed plant fragments without fiber (sugar, for example), often referred to as refined carbohydrates, can have detrimental health effects. As you can see in the table opposite, processed plant fragments have lots of carbohydrates, but almost all of them come from sugar or white flour. These types of carbohydrates are the forms most abundant in the standard American diet. Unfortunately, in the low-carb craze, the distinction between "good" carbohydrates and "bad" carbohydrates is usually forgotten.

One final thought about fiber. Fiber comes from things like the cell walls of plants and the tough coverings of plants. Fiber doesn't provide energy because we can't digest and break down and absorb all types of fiber, but it remains a crucial part of our diet. Only plants have fiber, and generally only whole plants have fiber. Processed plant fragments have often had all the fiber stripped away during processing. Fiber has a multitude of health benefits, but the only way to really get this vital nutrient is by eating unrefined fruits, vegetables, grains, and beans. I see so many patients with fiber-deficient diets diagnosed with diabetes, constipation, hemorrhoids, and many other diseases, and I'm amazed by how little people know about this wonder nutrient.

Minerals

In the table, the minerals are represented by calcium, iron, and potassium, although there are many others. How many times have you heard that to get calcium you must drink your milk? Or how many times have you been told that to get enough iron you must consume red meat? The fact is that as a *food group,* whole plants are, overall, far richer sources of beneficial minerals than animal foods are. There are individual exceptions, of course. Cow's milk has abundant calcium, for example. But in general, based on the food samples in the table on page 28, of the 10 minerals listed in the USDA's nutrient database (at http://ndb.nal.usda.gov, where these nutrient data came from), 8 of them are more bountiful in whole plants than in animal foods based on a calorie-to-calorie comparison. (Only three minerals are shown in the table.) Iron is more than two times more abundant in whole plants than in the animal foods! The only two minerals more abundant in animal foods are sodium and selenium. The poorest source of minerals, across the board, is the refined plant group. Some refined plant products, namely ready-to-eat cereals and enriched flours (neither listed in the table), are heavily fortified with a few minerals so the people who are subsisting on those foods do not become deficient in them.

Vitamins

The differences among the three food groups become even more dramatic when considering vitamins. In the table, vitamin C, folate, vitamin B_{12}, and vitamin A represent the vitamin group. Whole plants are the great factories of vitamins in nature. Some vitamins are thousands of times more abundant in whole plants than they are in any other food group, though some, including riboflavin, niacin, and pantothenic acid (not listed in the table), are certainly present in some animal foods even though they are not made by the animals. The only vitamin not present in plants is B_{12}. Microorganisms make B_{12} and it bioaccumulates in animal flesh. Humans require B_{12} in microscopic amounts (2 to 3 micrograms a day, equal to 5 to 6 *billionths* of a pound a day). Because of this requirement, I do suggest that those following a strictly plant diet take a B_{12} supplement (more on supplements in Chapter 11). Even with the B_{12} exception, the table makes it abundantly clear that to get vitamins, you must consume whole plants. Animal foods have mediocre amounts of some vitamins and are deficient in many. Refined plants are even worse. They are essentially devoid of vitamins. Again, commercial food processing has artificially supplemented some refined food products with vitamins, but make no mistake—the refining that is commonly done to plants strips them of their most valuable nutrients.

This small sample of vitamins does not include many nutrients known to be healthful, such as any of the multitudes of antioxidants and other phytonutrients that are thought to protect against many different diseases. These antioxidants are almost exclusively found in whole plants. The only antioxidants found in animal foods are those small amounts that the animal consumed and stored when it ate plants. They are present only in tiny, essentially negligible fractions compared to the amounts present in plants. Processed plant fragments are also deficient in antioxidants.

Let us not forget one final "nutrient": cholesterol. We do not have to consume cholesterol. Our livers can manufacture as much cholesterol as is needed for it to perform all of its vital functions in the body. In fact, cholesterol intake in the diet is known as something to be avoided due to the possibility that it will promote disease. Cholesterol is found only in animal-based foods. Just as fiber is present solely in plants, cholesterol is present solely in animal foods.

When looked at all together in terms of their macronutrient and micro-nutrient content (the latter including fiber, minerals, and vitamins), it is astonishing how different these three food groups are. The processed plant fragments are the most deficient of all. Processed plant fragments provide mostly "empty" energy without the crucial protein, minerals, or vitamins required for good health. The animal foods have mediocre amounts of minerals and vitamins—and several major deficiencies—but also have much more fat and cholesterol. The whole-plant food group is far and away the one with the complete package of beneficial nutrients: fiber, protein, minerals, and vitamins, including antioxidants, and they are low in fat and have no cholesterol. The only deficiency is in vitamin B_{12}.

The all-American diet is based on meat and processed plant frag-ments with minimal whole fruits and vegetables. Yet many describe their standard fare as a "balanced diet." Most patients I meet in the clinic or hospital consider their diet to be balanced. Those who consume mostly plants (including vegetarians or vegans) are often pressed about where they get their protein (or iron, or calcium, etc.). Questioners usually per-ceive these diets as imbalanced and warn that although it's okay to eat only plants, you had better be careful because you're at risk for nutri-tional deficiencies. But if you consume the whole-food, plant-based diet I advocate and you care about nutrients, it is clear that those who subsist on the traditional American diet are the ones at grave risk for nutrient deficiencies. I see it all the time in patients who come to the doctor's office with one or more chronic diseases: fiber deficiencies, minimal vitamin and antioxidant intake, excess cholesterol intake. These are the people eating the "balanced" American diet, and yet these are the people suffering from malnutrition. It's clearly time to reconsider what constitutes "balance."

THE THREE FOOD GROUPS IN DIETS

Now that you know how to divide foods into three food groups and some of the major nutrient differences between them, let us combine the food groups to create the optimal diet. I think the easiest way to describe the different dietary strategies is graphically. The pie charts that follow are schematics based on my own impressions. They are not based on actual survey data.

The standard American diet is heavy on meat, dairy, white flour, sugar, and oil. Imagine the standard fast-food meal of a cheeseburger, fries, and a milk shake. Or if you have a "healthy" American meal, you might have baked chicken, a side salad with ranch dressing, and flavored rice with beans. Whether it's the "healthy" version or the junk-food version, the standard American diet relies heavily on animal foods and processed plant fragments. The healthy version usually just substitutes less-egregious ingredients or preparation methods, such as having baked chicken instead of chicken-fried steak and using extra-virgin olive oil instead of lard. On average, an American eating this animal and processed plant fragment diet might be taking in something like shown in the Standard American Diet graphic opposite.

Whole plants sneak into the standard American diet as potatoes in the form of french fries, tomatoes in ketchup and pizza and pasta sauces, and perhaps one or two servings of fruits and vegetables a day. Otherwise the diet is primarily meat, dairy, and plant fragments. Think of the all-American foods: hot dogs with white flour buns, pizza, and macaroni and cheese.

Because this diet, along with our sedentary lifestyles, has made two-thirds of us overweight or obese, we've turned in droves to quick-weight-loss formulas and schemes. As I mentioned in Chapter 2, one of the more popular formulas recently has been the low-carb, high-protein diets such as the Atkins and the South Beach Diets. These diets might look something like the Low-Carbohydrate Diet graphic opposite.

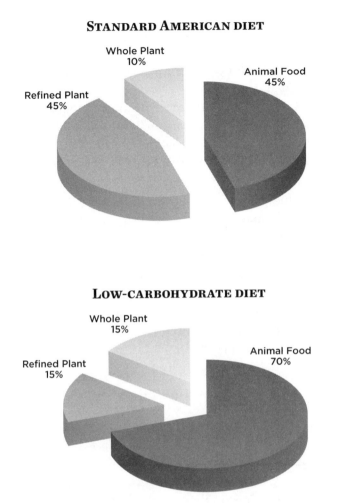

STANDARD AMERICAN DIET

Whole Plant
10%

Animal Food
45%

Refined Plant
45%

LOW-CARBOHYDRATE DIET

Whole Plant
15%

Animal Food
70%

Refined Plant
15%

Meals that are typical in this type of diet, especially during the strict early phases, might include a breakfast of eggs scrambled with cream and strips of fried bacon and then a lunch of grilled chicken and cheese, dark salad greens, and ranch dressing. The processed plant fragment portion of this diet would be 100 percent–fat products such as vegetable oil. The diet does not allow sugar or refined carbohydrates.

Swinging in the other direction, some people become vegetarians, avoiding all meat. However, most vegetarians consume large amounts of dairy foods. I know I used to. In fact, some vegetarians probably consume significantly more than the average amount as they replace meat with dairy-rich vegetarian foods. In terms of their overall nutrient content, there is little difference between dairy foods and meat. Dairy foods are comprised of high levels of animal protein and animal fat, cholesterol, minimal carbohydrates, and no fiber. The minerals and vitamins in dairy are somewhat unique (high calcium content, for example), but overall, since their nutrient profiles have more similarities than differences, dairy foods can be considered liquid meat. In one study of the vegetarian Seventh-Day Adventists,[2] almost 90 percent of the subjects who reported that they avoided eating all fish and meat still consumed dairy foods. In another large study in England,[3] people who described themselves as vegetarians had nutrient intakes that were surprisingly similar to those of self-described meat eaters. Fat, vitamin, and mineral intakes were roughly the same, and protein and carbohydrate intakes were only slightly different.[3] I can only infer that at least in terms of nutrients, the overall dietary intake of many vegetarians is not much different from that of a health-conscious meat eater due to vegetarians' high consumption of dairy, oil, sugar, and refined flour. Given these facts, the vegetarian diet pattern might look something like this:

VEGETARIAN DIET

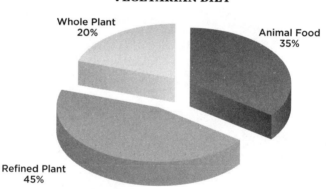

Whole Plant
20%

Animal Food
35%

Refined Plant
45%

Then there are vegans. They eat the vegetarian diet, but also avoid dairy and eggs and of course never eat any fish, fowl, or other meat. Some become vegan for their belief in the rights of animals and others become vegan for the health benefits. Many appreciate both. A vegan diet has in some studies been found to be consistent with excellent health. Vegans have consistently been found to be of a healthier weight and in one study had a 75 percent lower prevalence of high blood pressure and up to an 80 percent lower prevalence of diabetes.[4]

However, I am reluctant to simply embrace veganism as the optimal diet because there is a wide range of diets that fit vegan rules. "Vegan" by definition simply excludes all animal products. There is nothing about this definition that specifies what the diet actually should include. The crux of the matter is whether the animal foods are replaced with nutrient-depleted processed plant fragments or with whole plants. This is critical. It is in fact possible to have a vegan diet that is extremely unhealthy if animal foods are replaced with highly processed fake meats and fake cheeses, processed grains, sugars, and oils. Through the magic of food science it is increasingly possible to be vegan and actually consume fewer fruits and vegetables than a health-conscious meat eater. Given the wide range of dietary quality, the vegan diet is represented below by two different hypothetical compositions.

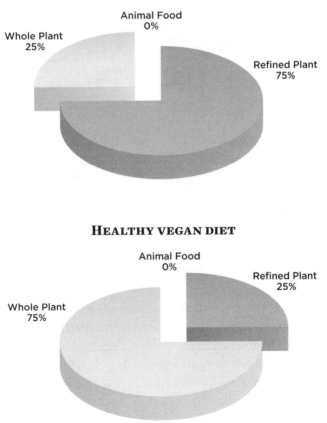

UNHEALTHY VEGAN DIET

Animal Food
0%

Whole Plant
25%

Refined Plant
75%

HEALTHY VEGAN DIET

Animal Food
0%

Refined Plant
25%

Whole Plant
75%

I don't know where most vegans fall on this broad spectrum, but I suspect it is somewhere in the middle, likely closer to the unhealthy version of a vegan diet. One recent study found that vegans consume amounts of fat similar to meat eaters, which can only mean they are eating plenty of added oils.[5] Every year I see more and more vegan foods in the grocery store that rely heavily on added oils, refined grains, and sugar.

So this brings us to what I think is likely the optimal diet: a whole-food, plant-based diet. This is the diet composed of the richest sources of nutrients. It is also the diet that's been shown to reverse heart disease and diabetes and to promote weight loss, among other benefits. It is based on whole grains, fruits, vegetables, and beans. It might look like this:

OPTIMAL DIET

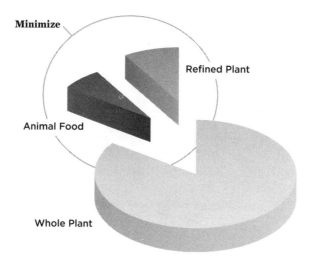

The small animal-foods portion of the diet allows for infrequent fish and seafood consumption or for lean meat to occasionally be used in very small amounts to flavor plant-based foods. The small bit of refined plant foods in the diet allows for use of practical conveniences that make it feasible for anyone to follow, such as some plain tofu, nondairy beverages like almond milk, and occasionally some sweeteners (maple syrup, sugar, fruit juice, etc.). We will talk more about what "minimize" should mean to you in the next chapter.

Simple enough, right? In theory, this is the simplest diet I know. In practice, I'll be the first to admit that going from the standard American diet to the optimal diet is a shift mentally, practically, and socially, and it demands a great change in habits and tastes. But it should now be clear where I believe your "goal line" should be. At this point, do not get bogged down in the details of the diet. As you will see, this optimal diet is far easier to practice than you may realize, and you'll be amazed by the new tastes of the foods you begin to eat. And this diet will give you the best health of your life.

Chapter 4

The Daily Practice

As you try to make healthy food choices, what does it mean to "minimize" animal foods and refined plants? Is it really that bad to eat a little bit of cheese (or chicken, or sweets, or whatever your favorite might be) here and there? Do you really have to go all the way?

Most people are concerned in particular about the prospect of totally giving up animal foods. I have to admit that as I consider types of healthy diets, I have my own uncertainties. As I mentioned in Chapter 2, I do not believe we are a vegan species. Traditional cultures around the world, even the most plant-based ones, with low rates of chronic disease and nonexistent heart disease, consume at least small amounts of animal foods infrequently. If you could eat the optimal diet from birth, I suspect that optimal diet might include *very small* amounts of fish, lean meat, or eggs as flavoring and infrequent meat-centered meals for special occasions (perhaps once a month or less). This would be in the context of minimal or no oil, sugar, or refined flour intake, moderate total calorie intake, abundant physical activity, and ultrahigh whole-plant-food intake.

The challenge I face as a doctor, though, is with patients who come to me after decades of eating junk—way too much animal foods and processed plant foods—whom I diagnose with diabetes, high cholesterol, high blood pressure, or obesity, or who perhaps I suspect have cancer or heart disease. Remember: If someone has been eating a typical American diet, trashing their arteries, for decades, I suspect they have some degree of heart disease. I know that their understanding of what are small amounts of animal foods, sugars, and oils is totally different from my idea of small amounts. Further, I know it can be difficult to make significant lifestyle changes if we do not draw bright lines in the sand as we plan our meals. If you have a little sugar at breakfast, just one cold cut at lunch, only one spoonful of oil dressing on your salad, a small chicken breast at dinner and only a taste of cake afterward, all of these small dalliances and tastes add up to a near-constant assault on your health. In some ways it actually is easier to communicate and follow a no-animal-foods, no-oils plant-based diet, and there is science to support the healthfulness of that approach. For those with advanced heart disease, for example, the only diet shown to reverse disease is one that prohibits almost all meat, most dairy, eggs, and added oils.

If you are exceptionally healthy and would like to know what small percentage of your diet may include animal foods or processed plants, we just do not know those details. There is not yet a great weight of evidence comparing a plant-based diet with small amounts of fish, for example, against a plant-based diet that avoids all meat. I cannot know whether having 3 ounces of fish or seafood at dinner once a week in the setting of an otherwise superb whole-plant diet will make any difference in your health. For the vast majority of diseases and measures of health, there simply has not been research to compare those who eat a no-animal diet to those who eat a low-animal diet.

Remember that dietary quality is not just about the animal foods. It also depends on the amount of refined plant fragments (oils and sugars and refined flours) that you eat.

Imagine, for a moment, the task of assessing the health of two patients based solely on their food diaries. One patient eats small amounts of meat (perhaps 2 ounces of chicken pieces once a week to flavor a casserole, soup, or rice dish), but otherwise is eating whole, unrefined plant foods almost exclusively. The other patient is 100 percent vegan but consumes daily coconut milk curries, fake meats and fake cheeses, vegan cookies and crackers, and enjoys sugary cereal in the morning. If I had these two patients and knew their food diaries, I would assume that the nonvegan was in better health than the junk-food vegan.

But while there are complexities and uncertainties in the science, I am going to suggest, as I do with all of my patients, that the goal should be to minimize—even eliminate—animal foods and processed plants in attempting a whole-food, plant-based diet. I do this not only because of some scientific evidence we do have, but also for practical considerations. You might be surprised to learn about the science of food addiction and how it affects our chances of successfully changing our diets.

THE SCIENCE SUPPORTING THE 100 PERCENT APPROACH

Even though it is not possible to say for sure that 100 percent plants is better than 95 percent plants, there is some evidence to suggest going all the way is more beneficial. The China Project, the research project carried out in the early 1980s, found that at the time, rural Chinese people had a diet totally different from the American diet. The rural Chinese diet was mostly plants and had relatively small amounts of animal foods. The animal-food portion of the diet ranged from very small to small.[1] They used meat more as a flavoring or for special occasions, and there was little or no intake of dairy foods in most areas. Interestingly, even within this range of low to very low intake of animal foods, there appeared to be a correlation between blood cholesterol levels and diseases of affluence as the animal-food intake increased.[1, 2] With diets that included even slightly more animal-based foods, cholesterol levels were higher, which in turn was linked to a greater prevalence of typical Western diseases.[1]

Other evidence relates to heart health. The most popular diet of moderation is the Mediterranean diet, which focuses on increased breads and cereals, fruits and vegetables, less red meat, more fish, less saturated fat, and more "healthy" oils like olive oil and rapeseed oil.[3] In the most famous Mediterranean diet study, it was indeed found to reduce the risk of heart attack or death in people with heart disease,[4] but they still experienced disease progression. There were almost as many people in the dietary treatment group who had elective heart surgery as there were in the standard care group.[4]

This effect has been shown in other trials as well. In one study,[5] several hundred heart attack survivors were divided into two dietary treatment groups. Both groups ate a mostly vegetarian diet, but one group ate far more fruits and vegetables. The group getting more fruits and vegetables had a lower risk of death and much less chest pain, but a full 25 percent of them, or one out of four, still had cardiac events (heart attacks, death from heart disease, etc.) within a year. This group was eating meat "only" a couple of times a week and eggs four or five times a week and was consuming "healthier" oils along with plenty of fruits and vegetables. Many people who advocate moderation would call that an ideal diet! With these moderate plant-based diets, the heart was becoming more diseased at a slower rate than with a diet containing fewer fruits and vegetables, but the disease continued in its sad march toward death.

Contrast these moderate Mediterranean diets with diets that have totally eliminated animal foods and added oils. Two doctors have documented reversal of blockages in the heart—Dean Ornish and Caldwell Esselstyn. Both have published research involving a whole-food, plant-based diet largely without animal products and no added oils. Patients that Dr. Esselstyn treated with this optimal diet, along with cholesterol-lowering medication, had the largest reversals of vessel blockages ever documented in the literature.[6] Dr. Ornish documented heart disease reversal with lifestyle alone, a cornerstone of which was the whole-food, plant-based diet.[7] And in a measure that's more important than the dimensions of a few blockages, Dr. Esselstyn's patients found that they avoided the signs of progression of disease, namely worsening symptoms, further surgeries, and death.[8]

Patients in these studies who adhere to the total diet *annihilate* heart-disease progression.

My rationale for recommending this way of eating goes beyond cardiovascular health. For those people concerned with other diseases, particularly cancer, I suggest going all the way, because it is quite possible that for dietary changes to make a difference in your outcome, you need to strictly adhere to an optimal diet. There is good evidence that diet is a key factor in cancer initiation and promotion, for example, but the results of some trials using moderate dietary changes have been disappointing. For example, eating a lower-fat diet by eating more baked chicken rather than steak or eating six servings of vegetables instead of four have not been shown to have much effect on cancer.[9-14] Moderate, small steps have failed.

BREAKING THE ADDICTION

What would the rate of successful smoking cessation be if I told patients who smoked that every time they avoided cigarettes Monday through Friday, they could go ahead and reward themselves with a couple cigarettes on Saturday night? From a health perspective this might be reasonable.

Does two cigarettes a week actually damage health for most people? I'm not sure. Two cigarettes a week would certainly be far healthier than a pack per day. But I would be the lousiest doctor ever. No one would ever quit smoking or even significantly reduce their smoking for any length of time if they rewarded themselves with a couple cigarettes every weekend.

As it turns out, some types of food aren't that different. There is more and more evidence that certain foods are addictive in the same way that drugs of abuse are addictive. It is theorized that in evolutionary times it was advantageous to have a taste system that favored the tastes of sweetness and fat so we would eat the ripe plants (the sweetest ones) and the foods with the most energy available given the cost of acquiring it (the fattiest foods). So our bodies reward us when we eat the sweet and fatty foods. What is the reward? Stimulation of the opioid and dopamine signaling pathways in our brains.[15, 16] These are the pathways that give us pleasure and reinforce our actions when we are doing things consistent with survival and perpetuating our species. These are the same reward systems hijacked in different ways by drugs like morphine, heroin, cocaine, nicotine, and alcohol. To this cast of bad actors we can now add highly refined pure sugar and fat.

One review[15] recently assembled a wide variety of research, mostly in rats, implicating sugar as an addictive substance. There are numerous characteristics of behavior related to sugar intake that are consistent with those seen with other highly addictive substances. When given the chance, rats increase their sugar intake over time (meaning they build tolerance and need a stronger stimulus over time). They binge on sugar meals. The sugar meals trigger the opioid reward pathway, a fact researchers have confirmed by giving the bingeing rats a drug that blocks the opioid system. These poor rats go into withdrawal and have "teeth chattering, forepaw tremor, and head shakes, as well as behavioral manifestations of anxiety."[15] Rats get anxious when you limit their access to the sugar diet, they get aggressive if you take away the periodic sugar treats, and they seek out sugar long after you take it away from them. Further supporting the idea that sugar is part of a powerful addiction system is that those sugar-bingeing rats who are forced to abstain increase their alcohol intake.

Hard-drinking rats may seem like a joke, but this is real research! In one of the more dramatic findings, when rats were given a choice to press a lever to get cocaine injected straight into their bloodstreams (which must be quite enjoyable!) or to press another lever to get a sweetened water treat, 94 percent of the animals preferred the sweetened water.[17] The researchers wrote:

> **As a whole, these findings extend previous research . . . by showing that an intense sensation of sweetness surpasses maximal cocaine stimulation, even in drug-sensitized and -addicted users. The absolute preference for taste sweetness may lead to a re-ordering in the hierarchy of potentially addictive stimuli, with sweetened diets (i.e., containing natural sugars or artificial sweeteners) taking precedence over cocaine and possibly other drugs of abuse.**

Findings also suggest that fat is an addictive substance, though there are some differences between fat and sugar addictions.[15] Unfortunately, fat may be more of a double whammy in that it was more likely to contribute to weight gain in these studies.[15, 18]

Knowing this, recognize that you may need to seriously limit or avoid these foods to break the addiction, just as many smokers need to give up all cigarettes to kick the habit.

BEGINNING THE DIET

Are you scared yet? It might seem like I am presenting an awful lot about trying to be perfect, but I don't want to give you the wrong impression. I want you to know that the optimal diet is likely to be a stricter diet, one that avoids the addiction cycles we fall into with the standard American diet. But I don't think you need to try to be perfect humans from day one and I don't want you to burden yourself with expectations of perfection.

I am simply defining the optimal diet. At the same time, I am suggesting that you give yourself the leeway to get there on your own terms.

No one is perfect, and if you have been eating the standard American diet your whole life, you know I am asking you to make one of the biggest lifestyle changes you have ever considered. Do not beat yourself up if you're not perfect from day one. When I counsel patients, I advise them to look at making a dietary or lifestyle change as an experiment. Keep a short-term, specific goal in mind. For example, do a 2-week trial with the help of this book and allow yourself the freedom to leave the rest of your life "up in the air." After 2 weeks, you can make a new decision. You can try the Paleo diet if you want, or the all-fast-food diet if you want, though I hope I've done my job better than that!

I find that if people think about making a change as a short-term commitment or experiment, it becomes far less daunting. If it's a short-term commitment, then the pressure is on me to convince you in just a couple of weeks that your life is going to be better this way. There's no pressure on you to make a major lifelong commitment to a perfection that you have to begin right this second.

The Building Blocks of Success

I want you to maximize your chance of success. There is a theory about behavior change called the self-determination theory. It states, among other things, that we all have basic psychological needs that are critical for motivation and personal well-being. If you can fill these needs, you'll do well. They may be the foundation of whether you succeed or fail. These are the three needs:

1. **Autonomy.** The need to feel in control of your own choices—you're the boss

2. **Competence.** The need to have the skills and capability to achieve your goals

3. **Relatedness.** The need to feel close to and understood by important people in your life

These are very similar to the factors predicting successful behavior change that I mentioned in the Introduction. Let's go through them one by one.

Autonomy is the need to feel in control of your own actions; it's the need to know that your choices are your own. How many times have you tried to make someone change and had it fail? How many times has someone tried to make you change? It doesn't work very well, does it? You're not going to succeed at change unless you feel like you are generating the change yourself. Complying with rules that have been pushed upon you to change a behavior provides weak motivation. It often doesn't work.

So as you embark on this dietary change, one of the most important actions you can take is to decide why you are doing this. If you have clear, personal reasons that motivate you and if you feel positive about the change, then you are in good shape. Positive thoughts are more powerful and motivating than negative thoughts or thoughts based in fear or misery. For example, embarking on this diet because you hate your body shape and think of yourself as a lazy slob (you think over and over, "Why can't I stick to a diet, anyway?") is a weak motivation, and any changes you do make likely won't last. In contrast, embarking on this diet because you love your family and others in your life, you love the activities you do, and you want your diet to support you in your efforts to enjoy these aspects of your life is a positive motivation, and it may be stronger and longer lasting. The best thing about this diet is that as you get further into it and conquer some of the challenges and reap some of the benefits, you will begin to know deep inside that you are moving in a positive direction. I have heard countless people say that once they made the change, it became self-reinforcing as they experienced more benefits.

Whatever your reasons, it is important that you make this change primarily for yourself. If you are being forced to read this book by your spouse, your child, or someone else, it's time for a gut check: Do you want to improve your life by improving your diet? If you do, can you name the reasons that are motivating *you* to change?

This is the bottom line: *This should be YOUR choice, and no one else's. If you don't really want to change your diet, then put the book down and think about coming back to it later, when you're ready.*

The need for **competence** is the need to feel capable, the need to feel that you have the skills to do this. Changing your diet is not easy and may involve significantly different skills than you are used to. How do you cook vegetables to be appealing? How do you cook anything? How do you read labels? What do you buy when you shop? Where do you eat out?

This book, particularly the last part of it, is intended to give you an introduction to those skills, and with a little practice and time you'll be on your way to having the confidence to succeed at changing your diet. The recipes in this book are taken from my favorite cookbooks and are for simple, fast, tasty dishes that anyone can make. After a 2-week trial with these recipes, along with the tips I'll give you to help you through the day, you'll have significant skills and confidence.

Here is a sample of the basic skills you'll need to get started. You can do this. Anyone can do this.

Reading Labels

I want to make this as easy as possible as you start navigating food shopping in a whole new way. When you pick up a packaged food in the grocery store, you can look at the Nutrition Facts label and get very confused very quickly. Let's simplify it: Right away, I want you to ignore the box with all the numbers and breakdowns of this or that nutrient.

Instead, I want you to look below the Nutrition Facts box to the list of ingredients. The list is ordered so that the first ingredient is the most prevalent one by weight. If there is 1 ounce of flour and ½ ounce of sugar in the food, the flour will be listed first, and then the sugar. By the time you get to the end of the list for many processed foods, you've reached the ingredients that are present in rather small amounts compared to the main ingredients of the food.

As you look at this list of ingredients, ask yourself these two questions:

1. Is this a whole food?

2. Is it a plant?

If most of the ingredients are whole foods, then you've passed step one. If you are eating a food with flour in it, be careful that you are getting 100 percent whole-grain flour. Sugars, sweeteners, and oils are not whole foods. The food is more or less of a whole food depending on how much of the product is made up of these food fragments.

The second question is whether it is a plant. This is usually an easy question to answer. If the ingredients are plants, you have passed step two. If the food passes both tests, it is likely a more health-promoting food. If it doesn't, put it back on the shelf and try again.

That's it. That's the basic approach I want you to use when you're navigating the grocery store. I'll offer you more advanced tips, particularly on figuring out how much salt, sugar, and fat are added to a food, but for now just focus on the ingredient list and getting foods that pass the two tests: whole food and plant. Do that and you're more than halfway there.

Like shopping at a grocery store, eating out can be difficult. We all love food that is tasty and convenient, but now that you are going to also eat for health, what should you order?

There are ways to eat out that are healthier, but I admit that it is difficult to follow a strict, optimal diet when you eat out. For people who are avoiding all oils to reverse heart disease, for example, eating out can be a rather treacherous, usually toxic activity no matter how hard you work to be "good."

What follows is a list of the types of foods that are safer than others when you eat out. This list is *not* consistent with optimal nutrition, and I recommend eliminating these processed foods as you find healthier alternatives, but when you're starting out, shifting the foods you get when you eat out can make a significant improvement in your health.

Somewhat Less Toxic Ways to Eat Out

FAST FOOD

Taco Bell: Bean Burrito, Fresco style (this modifier is often not easily found on the menu, but means that the cheese and dairy-based sauces are replaced with salsa)

7-Layer Burrito, Fresco style

Black Bean Burrito, Fresco style

Subway: Veggie sub without cheese. Get all the veggies (ask for extra!) and hold the mayo. Instead, try a little mustard with vinegar and oregano. None of the breads are perfect, but Honey Oat and 9-Grain Wheat may be marginally healthier than the others.

Burger King: If you're stuck at the fast-food burger place, try the veggie burger. Hold the mayo and get extra lettuce and tomato.

Local pizza joint or Papa John's: Cheeseless pizza with extra tomato sauce and all the veggie toppings

Breakfast: Some places have oatmeal made with water, including some fast-food restaurants, but be warned that any flavored oatmeal is going to be extremely high in sugar. Eating so much sugar in the morning isn't going to provide you with the long-lasting fuel you need.

SIT-DOWN RESTAURANTS

In general, you're going to find that the choices at the national chain restaurants become more and more boring as your palate expands. With your new diet, you will likely find a new world of ethnic foods at local restaurants.

Chinese: Many Chinese restaurants now have a "diet menu" offering a variety of steamed vegetables with sauce on the side. These can be very healthy (and tasty!).

Thai: Stick with vegetarian dishes and try to get as much steamed veggies as possible. This is tasty food, but beware of the curries, which are absolutely saturated with fat.

Indian: Like Thai food, you can get plenty of veggies in this food, but it often has added fat in the form of oil or ghee. Nonetheless, it is better than meals that don't have any vegetables.

Greek: Hummus, eggplant, grilled veggies. Minimize oils, if possible.

Mexican: Veggie fajitas, veggie burritos. Minimize oils, if possible, by ordering steamed veggies. Skip the cheeses and sour cream.

Ethiopian: There are lots of delicious flavors with veggies and beans in this food.

Italian restaurants: This used to be one of my favorite cuisines, but I have to admit I have become more and more bored with typical Italian fare. The vegetarian dishes are usually tasteless and unhealthy concoctions comprised of white flour, tomato, oil, and salt, but you can almost always find pasta primavera or spaghetti marinara.

Lastly, to succeed in this change you need to satisfy your need for **relatedness.** This means that you have social support from those people in your life that matter to you. This is crucial. I see over and over that this is the predominant factor deciding success or failure. It is very difficult for one person in a marriage, for example, to radically change their diet if their spouse is not supportive. Let those to whom you are close know why you are changing your diet and why this journey is meaningful for you. Ask if they would like to support you or even to participate in some way. If you can have a friend or partner take this journey with you, you will benefit in numerous ways. You will not only have emotional validation when you are having a hard time or feeling happy about a success, but also a partner who can help you hone your skills, acquire knowledge, and suggest new things for you to try.

If you feel alone as you consider taking this dietary journey, I urge you to make a serious attempt to find some source of social support before you begin. There are social groups focused on food in most cities. Consider attending a local vegetarian club outing, for example. Consider community wellness programs or even starting a wellness group at your church. If all else fails, there are apps and Web sites that provide virtual communities and support. In today's age of blogs, apps, and recipe databases, you're just an Internet search away from finding a wealth of information provided by a community of people who have also taken this journey.

INTO THE WILD

Believe it or not, you have now read enough information in this book to be well armed to take control of your health. You have some important, fundamental knowledge, including some understanding of and exposure to research linking diet to health. You know an entirely new way of thinking about food as the three food groups. You know what the goal is, the optimal diet. Furthermore, you know the most important building blocks to help you succeed. You understand your motivation, you know some fundamental skills, including the most important aspect, how to read labels, and you know how you can enjoy eating out. You know you must rally your social supports.

With all of this, you know vastly more than most people about nutrition and health and how to apply it in your life. Don't worry, though; you won't be sent into the wild just yet. In the next part of this book, we'll cover specific questions about the diet and areas of confusion. In the last part, we'll tackle the practicalities in much greater depth, and offer a 2-week menu plan with recipes. It can be used as a resource for trying different cookbooks or you can follow every word and embark on a 2-week experiment that will offer step-by-step instructions for making the most important health change of your life. By the end, you will be *expert* at improving your health and life through diet.

Part 2

HOT TOPICS

Chapter 5

Refined Plants: Sugar and Soy

One of my favorite radio advertisements is a dialogue between two truck drivers for two different soda companies. They meet in what seems like a truck-stop diner, and one proceeds to beg the other for a taste of some soda from the competing truck. In this effort he sounds like a hard-core stoner, desperate for his next hit of soda. They have a funny dialogue and finally the desperate man gets a taste of the other soda. He ends up guzzling the whole drink, much to the dismay of the other driver. It makes me chuckle every time because of how ridiculously badly the one driver needs to taste the other soda.

If you start to pay attention to food marketing, you will see this addiction motif everywhere. Whether it is in advertising or packaging and labeling, you will start to appreciate how common it is for companies to blatantly imply that you will become addicted to their food product. There is a sugar cereal called "Krave," a potato chip company that had the tagline "Betcha can't eat just one," and on and on. And guess what? The advertisers are right! They are addictive. These foods are technologically advanced mixtures of food fragments and chemicals that hijack our brains' reward pathways. They trick our outmatched primal brains into thinking we are consuming the right foods in order to survive and reproduce. They are sometimes called hyperpalatable foods. These foods, from the processed-plant food group described previously, make up the bulk of the plants consumed in America.

They are to be avoided. Mostly they consist of sugars, oils, and refined grain flours, but they also increasingly consist of soy products and isolated protein products.

SUGAR

Let us start with that not-so-glorious substance that is scientifically proven to be addictive and may come as white crystals or powder: sugar. I was doing an interview once, and the writer commented that out of the whole gamut of diets she had tried, the one thing that all of them have in common is the avoidance of sugar. This is an area where the plant-based advocates and the low-carb advocates can agree, which makes it very special and rare indeed. Added sweeteners come in many different forms and will show up on ingredient lists under many different names, as shown below.

DIFFERENT TYPES OF ADDED SWEETENERS

Glucose, galactose, lactose, fructose, dextrose, sucrose

Corn syrup, high-fructose corn syrup, rice syrup, maple syrup, agave syrup (marketed as "nectar")

Sugar (usually from sugarcane or sugar beets)

Honey

Dehydrated cane juice

Fruit juice concentrate

Artificial sweeteners: aspartame, sucralose, saccharin, neotame, acesulfame potassium, cyclamate

For Americans, like the lab rats, sugar appears to be highly addictive. Based on government nutritional surveys, a National Cancer Institute model finds that the average American 1 year of age and older consumes an astounding 22 teaspoonfuls[1] of added sugar a day, or about 345 calories[2] a day. Adolescents, especially males, take the cake—literally. Males ages 14 to 18 consume more than 34 teaspoons,[1] or about 530 calories,[2] of added sugars a day. Thirty-four teaspoons is almost three-quarters of a cup. This same group of males, like many other demographic groups, consumes about 1/100th of a cup of dark-green vegetables daily.[3] In other words, in terms of pure volume, they consume more than 70 times the amount of added sugar as they do dark-green vegetables.

By several measures, our intake of added sugars has increased significantly over the past 30 years.[4] We get anywhere from 11 to 20 percent of all of the calories we consume from added sugars, with younger Americans at the high end of the range and older adults at the low end.[5] The following table shows where we get our sugar.

PERCENTAGE CONTRIBUTION TO TOTAL INTAKE OF ADDED SWEETENERS, BY FOOD GROUP

Soft drinks	33%
Solid sugars/sweets (table sugar, honey, syrups, candies, jams, jellies, gelatin desserts)	16%
Sweetened grains (cookies/cakes)	13%
Fruitades/drinks (fruit punch, fruit juice drink, lemonade)	10%
Milk/milk products (chocolate milk, ice cream, sweetened yogurt)	9%
Other grains (cinnamon toast, honey-nut waffles)	6%

Source: Guthrie JF and Morton JF. Food sources of added sweeteners in the diets of Americans. *Journal of the American Dietetic Association* 2000;100:43–51.

Why does sugar matter? I think it is a threat to our health not necessarily because of what sugar *is,* but what it is *not.* Sugar is pure, high-density energy calories without any of the nutrients present in whole foods, such as vitamins, minerals, fiber, essential fats, or protein. As mentioned in the last chapter, it is highly addictive, and lab rats that binge on food containing sugar and fat consume more calories overall and gain more weight.[6] In humans, there is now evidence suggesting that we do exactly the same. Increased sugar consumption is linked with higher calorie consumption, obesity, diabetes, kidney stones, gallstones, cavities, increased blood pressure, blood cholesterol imbalances, and lower intakes of protein, fiber, and vitamins and minerals.[4, 7–12] The evidence is not strong enough to suggest that you must obsessively avoid all added sweeteners in all of your food, but you should avoid predominantly added-sugar foods (sodas, candies, pastries, and many cereals, as well as fruit-juice, sport, and energy drinks, for example). You will likely be far healthier in the long run. As with many of my recommendations, people struggling with weight problems, eating addictions, and diabetes may need to be far stricter.

Many people substitute artificial sweeteners for sugar. There are many varieties, such as those listed on page 53. These chemicals have highly potent sweetness but do not contain significant calories, so they are used to flavor soda with zero calories. Sounds great, right? Unfortunately, I must advise against consuming artificial sweeteners. An excellent review paper that was recently published[13] notes that several studies have now shown that intake of artificial sweeteners is correlated with weight gain over time. Interestingly, artificial sweeteners may increase both appetite and the drive for sweet foods. They trigger the food reward pathways in the brain without satisfying them the way real calorie-laden sugar does, thus possibly leading to increased calorie intake.[13] Imagine it this way: You have an afternoon diet soda drink and then at dinner you are a bit more interested in dessert than you would be if you had just had water earlier. In addition, people who practically subsist on diet drinks are likely to be forever held hostage to their need for sugary foods, partly due to the sweetness of their artificial sweetener intake. Skip the soda and skip the diet soda as well. Diet drinks are not a healthful alternative.

SOY FOODS

Another surprisingly common refined plant is the soybean. It yields products from oil to flour to tofu, which are totally different from sugar, of course, but they are everywhere. I always hear a lot of questions about soy foods and health, particularly from those people trying to reduce or eliminate their animal-food intake. Twenty years ago, there were very few soybean-based meat and dairy replacements available in most grocery stores. But as more and more people have adopted a plant-based diet, the availability of soy products has skyrocketed. There are many types of milks, cheeses, frozen desserts, and meat replacements made from soybeans. These products are also in prepackaged frozen meals like pizzas, burritos, and pastas. And while soy is one of the most prominent ingredients, many of these products instead use other types of refined flours, oils, or wheat protein.

These products allow people to eat a diet devoid of animals while still satisfying their taste preferences. This is very useful for those people who are just beginning to shift their diets to plant-based diets. It makes it possible to put your toe in the water and try some nonmeat foods without struggling to reinvent every taste bud in your mouth. In addition, even longtime herbivores find these soy products convenient and tasty, thus explaining their popularity.

My concern about many of these convenience soy products is the same as it is with other refined plant foods. Many of them are highly refined and have added oils or sugar. I encourage you to look at the ingredient lists of foods that mimic meat and dairy foods and notice that they often rely on oil and other highly processed food components. Unsurprisingly, they are often much higher in fat and lower in healthful micronutrients than the original whole-plant foods. While not a soybean product, one of the leading vegan cheeses, for example, currently gets more than 50 percent of its calories from fat. Its top four ingredients are water, flour, and different types of oils. This makes it a calorie-dense food that is deficient in many of the healthful micronutrients, as well as the protein, that are present in the original whole plants.

Phytoestrogens

One of the more common questions I am asked regarding soy specifically is whether the presence of phytoestrogens in soy foods is harmful or beneficial. Phytoestrogens are families of chemicals in food that have weak estrogen-like hormone activity. Soy foods are high in isoflavones, one of the families of phytoestrogens, so when you eat tofu or soy products, you get exposed to more phytoestrogens than you would by eating most other foods. Much of the confusion about this issue started when it was noted that Asian populations that consumed more soy foods had far lower rates of breast cancer. Of course there were all sorts of dietary differences between the populations, but because scientists found phytoestrogens in soy to be related to estrogen receptors in the body, research focused on these specific chemicals as a possible mechanism for the breast cancer differences.[14] In a way, it was a classic case of the naïve biological reductionism within our system that drives scientists to do work that will enable the creation of a product (a pill or supplement) that will make money. Phytoestrogens and their actions in the body are extremely complex and largely a mystery at this point. These chemicals have widely variable activity based on what they are eaten with, the environment in the intestines (what bacteria are present or absent), and the person's genetics and body size, to name just a couple of factors.[15] Some phytoestrogens act in opposition to the estrogen activity in the body and some work in concert with it.

The bottom line is that phytoestrogens are nutritionally unimportant. For all the pizzazz of the idea that estrogen-like compounds are in your food, these compounds are just several of thousands you eat every day. Your overall diet and lifestyle are far more important. Your overall diet has important ramifications for the estrogen hormones produced by your own body, which are far more active and far more important biologically than any phytoestrogens you might eat in your food. Studies have shown the bodies of both premenopausal and postmenopausal women make significantly less estrogen when eating low-fat diets,[16] which is likely to be far more important than the effect of any phytoestrogens. In the end, the Asian communities that were studied were far more likely to have lower breast cancer rates not because of their consumption of soy phytoestrogens, but because they were eating low-fat, plant-based diets and maintaining a healthy weight with an active lifestyle.

Phytoestrogens, even when given as supplements or as concentrated soy foods, have failed to show any reliable effects on menopausal symptoms.[17] They do not cause any statistically significant increase in hormone-related side effects, including breast cancer, uterine cancer, and vaginal bleeding,[18] and they do not affect male hormones,[19] nor is there good evidence that they affect male fertility.[20]

I believe we can leave the phytoestrogen confusion behind us knowing that phytoestrogens are unlikely to have a negative impact on our health. In fact, recent studies have continued to confirm a link between higher soy intake and improved breast cancer outcomes.

Looking at the whole picture, though, I do recommend avoiding regular servings of refined soy products, mostly because I want you to have a well-rounded diet with plenty of fiber, no added fat, and an abundance of micronutrients. You can eat edamame, or any whole soybeans, as much as you want. And a little bit of tofu a couple times a week as an addition to dishes rich in vegetables can be nice for variety and taste.

- The typical American diet is overloaded with added sugars.

- Added sugars, which come under many names, are empty calories, offering little nourishment. You do not need to obsessively avoid all added sweeteners, but definitely avoid all predominantly added-sugar foods (candies, pastries, sodas, and fruit and sport drinks and juices).

- Avoid artificial sweeteners.

- Processed soy products should be limited in an optimal diet. They may be useful for a short time period while transitioning away from a meat-based diet.

- Phytoestrogens in foods are not likely to be important compared to the estrogens made by the body.

Chapter 6

Oils and Fats

One of the greatest sources of confusion in the health community today is the role of various oils and fats in disease outcomes. The public has been barraged by mixed messages. The overarching theme in the past several decades has been that all fat is bad, with saturated fat being particularly dangerous. More recently, health experts have been questioning the low-fat-diet mantra and suggesting that it is not the *amount* of fat that matters, but instead the *type* of fat.[1] We have heard that unsaturated fats are healthier, especially the polyunsaturated fats. These polyunsaturated fats are billed as being not only less dangerous, but even health promoting.

Intertwined in this discussion is the aura of good health imbued by the Mediterranean diet. As the Mediterranean diet has become more popular, the reputations of olive oil and canola oil and other liquid plant oils have improved because that is what they use in the Mediterranean countries. Now these oils are commonly described as "heart healthy" and able to lower the risk of disease. Exuberance abounds for tasty, "good," and "healthy" oils. It sometimes feels as if we are being encouraged to liberally drink the healthy oils whenever we want. One recent food pyramid from Harvard University positions healthy fats and oils at the foundation of your diet, alongside fruits, vegetables, and whole grains.[2]

Wait a minute. What happened to the low-fat message? In fact, what happened to the saturated fat message? Most recently, we have heard that saturated fats are not as bad as we were once taught,[3] and it seems that coconut oil is suddenly more in vogue.

As if we were not confused enough, we also have heard that we must avoid trans fats at all costs because of the unique damage they do to the cardiovascular system. Corporations do not mind this message too much because they can use food-science magic to eliminate trans fats and then come out with promotional campaigns advertising their efforts to make their foods healthier, all without fundamentally altering the foods they sell. You may have heard of major fast-food chains taking steps to make their foods trans fat free.[4] Apparently, now we can relax and know that fried chicken, french fries, and high-fat, highly refined sweets are safe again. Can you sense my sarcasm?

In this mess we have been confused about the benefits (or is it dangers?) of margarine and butter. If you are working hard to follow the discussion, you might even worry about the respective "smoke points" of oils you use.[5] And is extra virgin better than virgin? What does that mean, anyway? Then there is the related topic of fish and fish oil consumption, encouraged because the flappy animals are a rich source of omega-3 fats. (I will address fish and omega-3 supplements more specifically in Chapters 7 and 11.) What are omega-3 fats?

All of this confusion manifests itself in widely varying popular diets. The Atkins Diet and other high-protein diets encourage unlimited fat consumption, whereas other diet books, including this one, advocate for a no-added-fat approach. Both approaches have been shown to cause weight loss in the short term.

The confusion is not limited to the public realm. There are plenty of confusing studies with inconsistent and contradictory results in the scientific world as well. Perhaps no nutrient or group of nutrients has gotten as much scientific attention as the different types of fat.

It is no wonder that this is one of the most confusing of all nutrition topics!

WHAT IS OIL?

In light of this muddled background, I would like to make it as simple as possible by beginning with this observation: All oils and pure-fat products are entirely unnatural. In nature, you will never stumble upon any repositories of edible oils or pure solid fats. There are high-fat foods like different types of seeds, the fatty parts of animals, and whole milks, but all of these have many other components beyond the fat. Pure bottled oils and packaged solid fats are man-made, chemically or mechanically refined components of whole foods that do not naturally exist in nature in this refined state. If you believe in evolution, you can easily grasp the concept that at no point in the evolution of our biological systems did our ancestors frequent puddles of olive, canola, or peanut oil to slurp down the fatty acids that are now considered heart healthy and health promoting. Yet somehow we made it to this point in history, and we did it with only whole foods.

Why is this important? Because if we place any importance on nutrients, it is obvious that unnatural pure-fat products have very few nutrients that we know promote health. And yet they are the most energy-dense foods known. It is the same as the pure-sugar products previously mentioned. The table below compares the nutrient contents of whole soybeans and soybean oil, whole corn and corn oil, and whole olives and olive oil.

NUTRIENT CONTENT OF 100 CALORIES OF SOYBEANS, CORN, AND OLIVES* AND THEIR REFINED OILS

	SOYBEANS, RAW	SOYBEAN OIL	SWEET YELLOW CORN, RAW	CORN OIL	OLIVES, RIPE, CANNED*	OLIVE OIL
Protein (g)	8.8	0	3.8	0	0.7	0
Total fat (g)	4.6	11.3	1.6	11.3	9.3	11.3
Carbohydrates (g)	7.5	0	21.8	0	5.4	0
Fiber (g)	2.9	0	2.3	0	2.8	0
Calcium (mg)	134	0	2	0	76	0
Iron (mg)	2.4	0	0.6	0	2.9	0.1
Sodium (mg)	10	0	17	0	639	0
Vitamin C (mg)	19.7	0	7.9	0	0.8	0
Vitamin A (IU)	122	0	217	0	350	0
Saturated fats (g)	0.5	1.8	0.4	1.5	1.2	1.6
Monounsaturated fats (g)	0.8	2.6	0.5	3.1	6.9	8.2
Polyunsaturated fats (g)	2.2	6.5	0.6	6.2	0.8	1.2

*Nutrient data for raw olives was not available, so canned olives were used.

Source: USDA National Nutrient Database for Standard Reference, Release 24.

Soybeans are incredibly nutrient-rich foods. One hundred calories of raw soybeans has abundant protein and fiber and a wide variety of good vitamins and minerals that are nicely packaged with a good balance of fats. A quarter cup of raw green soybeans has as much calcium as about a half cup of 2% milk. Soybean oil, on the other hand, has had almost every good nutrient stripped away, providing you with nothing but pure fat and ultra-concentrated calories. Corn is just a lowly grass, but it also is surprisingly nutrient rich. It has more than adequate protein, fiber, and several minerals and vitamins. Again, all of this is lost when corn oil is made. And finally, even the fatty, salty canned olive has redeeming nutrients, including fiber, calcium, iron, and vitamin A. You would have to eat more than half a pound of ready-to-cook raw turkey (yielding 200 grams) to get as much iron as is found in 10 tablespoons (87 grams) of these olives. Or you could guzzle a whole glass of olive oil and be iron deficient.

The simple table on page 61 makes it clear that these unnatural food-industry products that we buy as pure fat in jars, bottles, and cans from a grocery store shelf are severely nutrient-deficient, isolated fractions of real food.

It is worth taking some time to explain calorie density in a bit more detail. "Calorie density" is a term used to describe the number of

CALORIE DENSITY OF VARIOUS FOODS
IN COMPARISON TO OLIVE OIL

To consume as many calories as there are in 1 tablespoon of olive oil (119 calories), you need to eat one of these:

4½ cups cherry tomatoes

12 cups shredded iceburg lettuce

17 cups raw spinach

3 cups cooked spinach (boiled and drained)

Almost 4 cups raw broccoli

More than 2 cups cooked broccoli (boiled and drained)

⅔ cup baked sweet potato

A bit more than ⅓ cup dry cereal oats

⅔ cup cooked whole-wheat spaghetti

Source: USDA National Nutrient Database for Standard Reference, Release 26.

calories in any given volume of food. Most people do not realize how energy dense oil and fat products are compared to real foods. A classic example of this misunderstanding that I see over and over is people thinking they are being healthy by eating a salad, but it is made up of some greens, two or three pieces of vegetables, croutons, cheese, and perhaps ham or chicken, all topped off with an oil-based dressing. Make no mistake, this is a fat- and animal-based meal. Only a tiny portion of the calories will come from unrefined plants. Most unrefined plants are very low in calorie density. The meat and fat are far more calorie dense. The table on the opposite page shows how many whole-plant foods you have to eat to get as many calories as there are in just *1 tablespoon* of olive oil.

As you can infer from the table, raw vegetables are naturally very low in calories, due largely to their high water content. Cooked vegetables are more energy dense because they have lost their water, but they still are not what you would ever call energy-dense foods. High-starch plants (potatoes and various grains, for example) are naturally more energy dense, but even these do not come even remotely close to the energy density of oil. You can make a huge salad, and as soon as you put a couple tablespoons of oil-based dressing on it, most of the calories from the meal will be coming from pure, refined fat. The take-home message is that you can make a wide variety of meals using whole-plant foods, and the minute you add any oil, the calorie content will spike *very* quickly and the calories will be coming from man-made, severely nutrient-deficient food fraction products.

THE SCIENCE BEHIND THE CONFUSION

In defining pure-fat products, I have obviously painted a simplistic, negative picture. Yes, oils are deficient in the good nutrients found in the original whole-plant food, and yes, oils are ultra calorie dense. But why are some oils widely praised and their use encouraged despite these obvious facts that are known by all experts? What am I not telling you? What is the science behind this topic, and why do the experts recommend certain fats?

This story begins 40 to 50 years ago, when a consensus was starting to build that dietary fat intake was one possible cause of breast cancer.

There were two lines of evidence: animal studies and human studies. Both were showing similar results. Observational studies showed that human populations with higher fat intake had higher rates of breast cancer. Animal studies showed that when you gave rats a known cancer-causing chemical and fed them varying levels of fat, higher-fat diets caused more tumor growth.[6] The human observational results supported what could be replicated in the lab. (Interestingly, the findings showed that polyunsaturated fats—the "good" fats that are currently in vogue—were more effective at promoting cancer in laboratory animals than saturated fats were.[6,7]) The same convergence of data was appearing with regard to colorectal cancer, as well.[7] In addition, prostate cancer, testicular cancer, ovarian cancer, uterine cancer, and pancreatic cancer were shown to be more common in populations consuming higher-fat diets.[7] Along with these cancer data, there was a growing body of evidence suggesting that high-fat diets were causally related to heart disease.[8,9]

All of this led to a growing concern that fat was the bad actor in the American diet. The capstone of the wave of research against fat was a 1982 blockbuster report called *Diet, Nutrition, and Cancer* from the US National Research Council that recommended lowering fat to 30 percent of total calories from the then-average 40 percent.[7] The committee that produced the report suggested that the evidence could justify a recommendation for an even greater reduction in fat intake, but they wanted to set a practical goal that people might actually achieve, so they somewhat arbitrarily suggested an upper limit of 30 percent.

From the early 1980s on, the low-fat mantra grew and became one of the most easily understood and recognizable features of nutritional recommendations. But as is usually the case, the research on fats and both cancer and heart disease had been more nuanced than what was commonly reported in popular culture. Not all types of fat seemed to be the same.

A Lesson in Fatty Acids

Based on the chemical structure of the fatty acid molecule, there broadly are two types of naturally occuring fatty acids, saturated and unsaturated (see the figure on the opposite page). The unsaturated fatty acids are comprised of monounsaturated fats and polyunsaturated fats, which also are distinguished by their chemical structures. In the polyunsaturated fat group are two types of essential fatty acids that humans must consume in their diet. We can synthesize all other types of fat, but we cannot synthesize these fatty acids, so they must be consumed. These two essential fatty acids are omega-3 and omega-6 fats. From these there are several types of derivative fats, including docosahexaenoic acid (DHA), eicosapentaenoic acid (EPA), and arachidonic acid, some of which might sound familiar to you. The omega-3 and omega-6 fatty acids are vital components of cell structures and processes and serve many vital functions in the body.

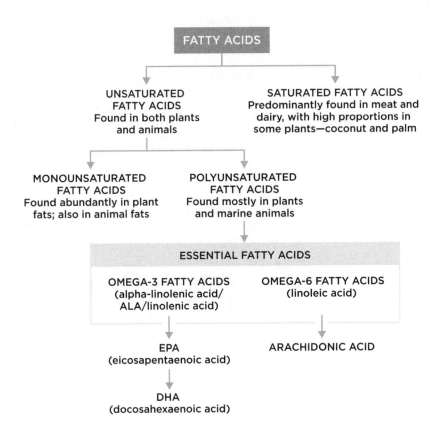

SEPARATING THE FATS

Several decades ago, scientists were questioning whether to value these different types of fats differently. At about the time that research implicating total fat intake in heart disease was accumulating, researchers noticed something a little strange in the native Inuit peoples in northern Greenland. By several reports,[10] these Inuit groups ate lots of protein and fat. Their traditional diet consisted of lots of marine meats, including fish, seabirds, and sea mammals. Yet at the time, based on weak evidence,[11] the Inuit appeared to maintain better cardiovascular status with less heart disease than Europeans.[12] How could this be?

It was postulated that their health might be better because their diet had a very high proportion of unsaturated fats, especially the essential omega-3 fats.[13] The research on the Inuit was very limited, though, and it didn't offer answers to any questions about fat as much as it generated questions. (As a point of interest, the early claim of lower rates of heart disease has been challenged with a thorough review that found the Inuit to actually have no less cardiovascular disease than comparison white populations.[11])

At about the same time that the anomaly of the Inuit was being explored, Ancel Keys, PhD, was completing his landmark research called the Seven Countries Study. He found that populations consuming higher levels of saturated fat compared to unsaturated fat had higher death rates and higher coronary heart-disease rates.[14] In other words, the populations eating nonmarine animals and dairy had higher death and coronary heart-disease rates than the populations who consumed more fish along with plant foods and plant oils like canola oil.

These findings, along with those of many other studies, set scientists off on a frenzied quest over the next 30 years to better understand the effects of different unsaturated fats, especially with regard to heart disease, but also with regard to cancer. There are very few nutrients that have received as much scientific attention as the different unsaturated fats have.

Two themes emerged:

1. Several (but not all) studies have shown that people who consume more unsaturated fats, and especially the omega-3 fats found in fatty fish, have lower rates of cardiovascular disease and mortality than do people consuming standard Western diets.[15–18]

2. The Mediterranean diet, richer in unsaturated fats and plants and

including less red meat and dairy, is linked to improved outcomes in cardiovascular disease, cancer, and neurodegenerative diseases like Alzheimer's and mild cognitive impairment when compared to the standard Western diet.[19, 20]

When you look at the whole story as it evolved over time, from the Inuit research to the modern Mediterranean diet research, it seems that a nice, consistent picture emerges: It seems that unsaturated fat is healthier than saturated fat. In fact, enthusiasm for unsaturated fats has dominated headlines. When people hear about the benefits of the Mediterranean diet, they hear about eating more olive and canola oils. This is no accident. Now the authorities can tell people to eat as much fat as they want as long as it is the appropriate type. This is a popular message that makes everyone happy. Most major health recommendations now include using various plant oils rich in unsaturated fats, as well as consuming foods high in essential fatty acids, namely fish. Olive oil and canola oil and other plant oils are depicted as heart-healthy foods to be widely and aggressively promoted.

I have a problem with this. There is some evidence that the unsaturated fats, especially the polyunsaturated omega-3 and omega-6 fats, are healthier than saturated fats. There is also a convincing, growing bank of evidence that the Mediterranean diet, relatively rich in plant oils, leads to improved health outcomes compared to the standard Western diet. *But these facts together do not lead to the conclusion that pure refined plant oils like olive oil are heart-health-promoting foods.*

Evidence that diets containing unsaturated fats *may* be healthier than high-saturated-fat diets

+

Evidence that the Mediterranean diet (higher in fruits and vegetables, fiber, and unsaturated fat and lower in dairy and red meat) is healthier than typical Western diets

≠

Edible plant oils are healthy.

THE MEDITERRANEAN DIET:
ANOTHER PERSPECTIVE

What is commonly left unspoken in many of these discussions is the fact that the Mediterranean diet is much closer to a vegetarian diet than the standard Western diet, having less meat and far less dairy. People who eat more fish and more of the polyunsaturated fats (certain plant oils) often eat more fruits and vegetables and less meat and dairy.[21, 22] In some studies of fat, these other aspects of the diet are not even considered.[16] So when someone touts the Mediterranean diet, we can't know if the benefits are because of the olive oil and fish or because of the increased plant-food intake and decreased meat and dairy intake. Could it be something other than the oil?

In one recent study, people that were asked to consume more olive oil had a slightly lower rate of stroke compared to people eating a high-fat diet,[23] but results from other studies on certain unsaturated fats have been less than sterling. For example, it initially seemed that fish oil lowered mortality after a heart attack.[24] However, a longer-term study[25] of men who had recently suffered a heart attack showed that eating more fish or taking fish oil is actually linked to an *increased* risk of cardiac death over a longer period of time. Yet another study of people with high cholesterol who supplemented with the omega-3 fat EPA showed reductions in several outcomes related to cardiac disease, but no difference in overall mortality or death from heart disease.[26] Other recent large summarizing studies combining data from many trials have shown there to be no significant benefit from fish oil for people with or without heart disease.[27, 28]

When all is said and done, despite all the vigorous enthusiasm for unsaturated fats, I do not believe you are going to improve your health significantly by using liberal amounts of plant oils or other fat supplements. In fact, I remain concerned that refined fat intake is not only unnecessary, but actually may be harmful. It is possible that the Mediterranean diet is healthy *despite* the added oil rather than because of it. The much greater emphasis on unrefined plants and lower animal-foods consumption is likely to be the most important aspect of the Mediterranean diet. One paper[29] with data all the way back to 1977 showed that across 40 countries, the coronary-heart-disease death rate among males ages 55 to 64 was most strongly linked to the intake of animal foods.

Interestingly, there were other areas of the world that had even lower heart-disease death rates than France and other Mediterranean countries. In rural China in the mid-1970s, where they were eating mostly plant foods without added oils, there were counties with hundreds of thousands of residents that had *zero* cases of death from coronary artery disease in people under the age of 65.[30] France during that decade had coronary death rates of about 200 per year per 100,000 men ages 55 to 64.[29] If you were from one of those counties in rural China in the 1970s, you might have wondered, "Why are the French people so ravaged by heart disease?" Could it be the high fat consumption? It seems plausible, as we know that within both Greece and Italy, people consuming more unsaturated fats have higher body weights.[31, 32]

In fact, we now know that there is an immediately negative effect on the body's blood vessels after exposure to fat. In a small study of obese people, subjects were given fat by IV infusion (commonly done in hospital settings) or given fat to consume by mouth.[33] These fats were mostly "healthy" unsaturated fats. Within hours these people had higher blood pressure, a higher heart rate, and poorer blood vessel function. Their arteries could not dilate as well as they had before the fat exposure, and the ability to dilate is a critical element of blood vessel function and health. Impaired arterial dilation has been shown to be a major risk factor for cardiovascular disease.[34–37] One study compared the consumption of a higher "healthy fat" diet (allowing lots of polyunsaturated fats) for 90 days to consumption of a moderately lower fat (and higher vegetable content) diet, and the blood vessels of the subjects eating the lower-fat diet were far better able to dilate.[38] Several other studies have shown relative blood vessel dysfunction after a *single* high-fat meal.[39–42]

And finally, back in 1990 researchers examined the heart arteries of men with known heart disease. They found that over 2 years, the men with the highest total fat intake—of polyunsaturated fats, specifically—developed new blockages in their hearts.[43]

In summation, one way to make sense of what seems to be a complicated mess of data is to think of this whole discussion as a matter of perspectives. If we compare the Mediterranean diet to the high saturated fat, meat, and dairy Western diet, we find it is consistently better for a variety of health outcomes. But what if we compare a no-oil, whole-food, plant-based diet with the high-fat, high-oil, plant-rich Mediterranean diet?

There are fewer of these studies, but the most convincing scientific results to date in my mind have come from trials in which patients with heart disease avoid every last drop of added oil along with fish, meat, and dairy. These studies have demonstrated the most significant reversals of heart disease ever shown.[44-47] Taken together with the other evidence that added oils, even plant oils, actually damage the cardiovascular system, it seems that the enthusiasm for olive oil and canola oil in the popular press is seriously misguided.

To my patients, I suggest leaving the confusion behind and getting back to the basics. Understand that edible oils and fats are highly refined, nutrient-depleted food fragments. They are the most calorie-dense food fragments you can consume. Stick with whole foods. For those with heart disease, this recommendation becomes extra important. I have no option but to recommend what has been shown to strikingly halt or reverse heart disease, and that is a strictly no-oil diet. How could I recommend less?

THE BOTTOM LINE

- Oils and solid fats are the densest foods available. You will consume more calories from a couple of tablespoons of oil than you will from a heaping pile of raw vegetables in your salad.

- Oils and solid fats are highly refined food fragments that are deficient in the good nutrients of the original food.

- Through time (at least until recently), unsaturated fats—particularly the essential fatty acids, including omega-3 fats—have been touted as being healthier than saturated fats.

- The Mediterranean diet is better than the standard Western diet for a variety of health outcomes, but perhaps worse than some diets that are mostly plants and no added oils.

- The most successful heart-disease-reversal diets are those that strictly avoid added oils.

- Taking everything into consideration, I recommend avoiding added oils and solid fats of all kinds.

Chapter 7

Fish

I come from a line of countryfolk and farmers who all fished regularly. As I was growing up and enjoying outdoors activities with my older siblings, fishing was commonly integrated into camping trips and canoe trips. My Granny Campbell was probably one of the best, most dedicated older fisherwomen on the East Coast. On family beach vacations through her eighties, she enjoyed nothing more than when we helped her to the end of an ocean pier or the edge of a pond so she could fish all day—even to the point of becoming sick from sun exposure.

I was never even half as skilled. I enjoyed hooking fish from a pond or river as a kid, but even then I was ambivalent, at best, about their smelly, slimy, scaly bodies, poopy guts, and button eyes that looked as though they might just have been pasted on. Gross! And I admit I also felt pretty bad for them because they thought they were going to get a nice, tasty worm but instead got a giant, sharp metal hook piercing the side of their face, sometimes through the eye socket.

To further my childhood problems, I never truly enjoyed the taste of fish. Though I have experienced the full culinary gamut, from savoring meat loaf, sausage, and scrambled egg and mayonnaise sandwiches during my childhood to loving my plant-based diet today, I never looked forward to eating fish. I did like the fried fish sandwiches of a certain fast-food chain (the one with the name of a clan in Scotland that was the Campbell clan's greatest enemy), but I think that was mostly because of the fried breading and tartar sauce. Similarly, I liked tuna sandwiches, but that was probably mostly because of the mayonnaise.

According to lots of organizations, I was on the wrong side of things. Siding with my granny, our national health and disease organizations are pretty high on fish. As a result, fish has become increasingly popular from a nutritional point of view. The American Heart Association recommends eating at least two servings of it a week.[1] As mentioned in the last chapter, fish is almost always praised for the merits of its fat content. Fish, especially certain types of fatty fish, are good sources of omega-3 fats, including EPA and DHA. Throughout the past several decades, a number of studies have shown that populations eating more fish have lower rates of cardiovascular disease.[2-9]

But this is far from the whole story. Investigating the effects of any one food or food group in the context of human diet and lifestyle is very tricky business. People are complicated, and we ingest thousands of different food chemicals that affect health in a synergistic way. It is difficult to do nutrition studies because it is amazingly difficult and expensive to measure people's average food intake accurately. At best, we can only somewhat accurately measure specific dietary components, including all different kinds of meats, dairy, processed foods (including sugar and oil consumption), as well as fruit and vegetable consumption. Then we have to wait 10, 20, 50 years for people to get chronic disease and die from it. At that point, trying to say that "Yes, this chronic disease is due to one nutrient or one food" is a naïve, difficult, and not a terribly defensible proposition. As a result, knowing for sure what effect any one food item or component will have on chronic diseases over the course of decades is difficult. This is true for fish, as well as for nuts or any other small food group. That's why we get so many conflicting headlines about single food items. We've all heard at one time that coffee is bad for us, then heard that it can be good. We've all heard that chocolate is bad, and also heard that it can be good.

What nutritional science can do well, however, is study larger dietary patterns. For example, we can look at overall dietary patterns in terms of general plant- versus animal-food consumption and more reliably assess their impact on chronic disease. We aren't trying to pick one factor out of thousands, but rather synthesizing thousands of individual factors into a pattern. In this way, we can be more confident that any associations we might find are real.

I mention this all as background to help you understand why we have had so many confusing studies about fish.

Interestingly, people who eat more fish may eat more fruits and vegetables and undertake greater physical activity. That makes sense, at least in societies such as ours. People likely eat fish instead of other animal foods. They do not likely substitute fish for vegetables. Increased fish intake has been associated with increased fruit and vegetable consumption, less meat consumption, or increased activity in studies from the United States,[5, 10, 11] Denmark (increased activity),[12] Finland, Italy, the Netherlands,[13] Japan, and Brazil.[14] Many of the studies[3] that have observed that increased fish intake is linked to decreased heart disease do not even measure these other diet and lifestyle factors, let alone try to take them into account when making assumptions about fish consumption. So is it possible that the benefit of fish consumption seen in some of these early studies was due to a combination of multiple good lifestyle choices, and not just fish intake?

IS OMEGA-3 ENTHUSIASM JUSTIFIED?

Furthermore, omega-3 fats, the fats abundant in some species of fish, do not appear to be the pure health bonanza that many have believed them to be. A large review[15] that was recently published combined the results of all the intervention trials investigating the benefits of omega-3 fats. The researchers found that increasing omega-3 fats by increasing foods high in omega-3 or taking a daily omega-3 supplement, no matter what the dose, did not significantly improve the rate at which patients died from any cause, how many heart attacks they had, or how many strokes they had.[15] If there is any effect of supplements, it seems it's that increased omega-3 fats may lead to improved outcomes for heart disease, but possibly worse outcomes for stroke. Another recent study[16] aggregated data from three large US studies looking at omega-3 fatty acid intake from fish consumption and rates of type 2 diabetes. Surprisingly, they found a clear relationship between increasing omega-3 fatty acid consumption and rates of diabetes. The people consuming the most omega-3 fatty acids had about a 25 percent increased risk of getting diabetes.[16]

In addition, much has been made of the anti-inflammatory properties of omega-3 fats.[17, 18] There are many studies indicating that omega-3 fats, especially when compared to omega-6 fats, can improve certain biochemical markers of inflammation.[18] There is some minimal evidence[17] that omega-3 fat taken as a supplement has mild benefits in rheumatoid arthritis, a disease characterized by inflammatory processes that have gone out of whack. But when researchers recently looked at critically ill people who were in an intensive care setting with acute lung injury, the results were very different.[19]

Acute lung injury, often called acute respiratory distress syndrome, is a severe, life-threatening cascade of inflammatory processes in the lungs most often related to severe infection, leading almost uniformly to patients requiring mechanical ventilation (being hooked up to a breathing machine) to survive. Researchers gave people on ventilators for acute lung injury omega-3 fats, one other fatty acid, and antioxidants as supplements and measured the outcomes. The trial[19] was stopped early because the patients who were getting the "anti-inflammation" cocktail were requiring more time on mechanical ventilation and more time in the intensive care unit; they experienced more days of diarrhea and they died at a higher rate. All of the anti-inflammatory cocktail's components had previously been shown to reduce inflammation in lab studies of intermediate inflammatory processes, things like immune cell signaling chemicals. Yet the patients receiving the cocktail were dying at a greater clip! This was an important trial, at least for acute lung injury, because in contrast to all the research looking at omega-3 intake's effects on one or two specific biomarkers like levels of immune system signaling chemicals, this trial actually looked at results that matter to patients: quality and length of life. The unequivocal result: The supplements were harmful.

Not Just Omega-3s

And what about the other nutrients in fish? Fish is essentially comprised of protein and fat, with some minerals (in smaller quantities than is found in many vegetables) and a couple of vitamins in significant quantities, but otherwise, it has minimal vitamin content. In addition, it has cholesterol and environmental toxins.

How about fish protein? As it turns out, fish protein may have health effects similar to those of other animal proteins. As a group, animal proteins are much more similar to each other than they are to plant proteins. The converse is also true: Plant proteins act much more like each other than they do animal proteins. This was well illustrated in a series of experiments[20] on rabbits. These rabbits were fed a low-fat, low-cholesterol diet with different types of proteins for 28 days and then their cholesterol was measured. As you can see in the graphic on page 76, though there are significant differences within the groupings of animal and plant proteins, they cluster together in rather dramatic fashion.

If fish protein is indeed similar to other animal proteins and we know that eating excess animal protein can cause mischief (higher blood cholesterol levels, increased kidney damage, poorer bone health, to name a few types of mischief), what are we to conclude about fish protein? It makes me a little less high on fish. We might be concerned about not only the effects of fish protein, but also the dietary cholesterol we get when we eat fish. Of course, we have long heard that lowering our cholesterol intake is a worthy goal. You will not be avoiding cholesterol by eating fish.

Finally, fish has one other problem that gets a lot of press: environmental toxins, specifically mercury. Mercury pollution in the environment becomes concentrated in fish, especially in fish that live for a long time and eat lots of other fish (sharks, for example). Increased mercury intake has been linked to an increased risk of heart attacks.[21, 22] In addition, mercury toxicity has been linked to neurologic symptoms in adults as well as significant neurologic development problems in children who were exposed to high doses of it in the womb through their mothers' diet, though there is much more limited evidence that the low doses commonly consumed in food cause these same problems.[23] These negative effects on health versus the benefits gotten with omega-3 fats are at the root of the abundant confusion over how much fish one should eat. Since fetuses are sensitive to environmental toxins via maternal exposure, special recommendations about fish consumption are made for pregnant women.[24] It all turns out to be phenomenally confusing because of what feels like inadequate science. That's because of what I mentioned earlier, the challenges of studying one chemical or food among tens of thousands of diet and lifestyle factors and trying to pinpoint the causes of health problems that take decades to develop. It can be an exercise in frustration.

I do not think anyone looking at the mountain of research can strongly advocate any specific conclusion with certainty. There has been a lot of evidence, although it is inconsistent, that people consuming more fish have a somewhat lower risk of heart disease.[1, 3, 23, 25, 26] In addition, early research identified specific ways in which the omega-3 fats found in fish might actually improve factors that put you at risk for developing cardiovascular disease.[1] However, much of the observational research (studies that simply observe fish intake and disease outcomes), the results of

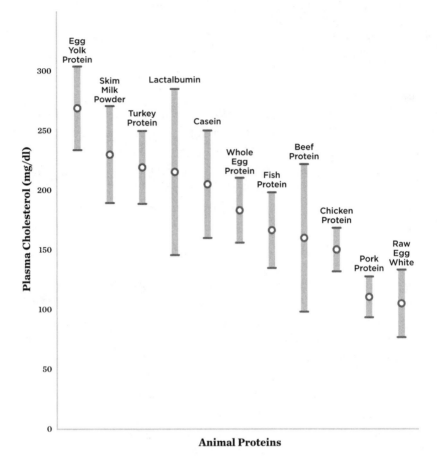

EFFECT OF DIFFERENT PROTEINS
ON SERUM CHOLESTEROL IN RABBITS

Source: Carroll KK. Dietary proteins and amino acids—Their effects on cholesterol metabolism. In: Gibney MJ and Kritchevsky D, eds. *Current topics in nutrition and disease, volume 8: Animal and vegetable protein in lipid metabolism and atherosclerosis.* New York: Alan R. Liss, 1983.

which have been inconsistent, has been seriously compromised by the researchers' failing to take other dietary factors into account. In addition, the enthusiasm for omega-3 fatty acids is lessening because of the more recent research that has shown a lack of benefits from its intake.[15] Perhaps most contrary to the push for fish consumption is that, as was the case with added oils, the most dramatic heart-disease reversal ever documented was accomplished with a diet that did not include fish or fish oil (though plants rich in omega-3 fats, like ground flaxseed, were used).[27]

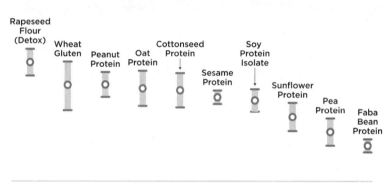

Plant Proteins

The frustrating truth is that I cannot say for sure if eating small amounts of fish (3 to 6 ounces per week) will make you healthier, make no difference in your health, or make you sicker. I do know that you do not *need* fish to thrive. On the other hand, however, significant data do link fish consumption with improved health. We know, for example, that some of the world's healthiest populations consume small amounts of fish regularly.[28]

For those who choose to consume fish in moderation (3 to 6 ounces per week), I recommend that you choose your fish and cooking method with care. The table below will help you choose a fish that is rich in the omega-3 fats while low in mercury, and it should be prepared without any added oil; instead, steam or bake it in parchment paper. Don't eat fried fish, and don't consume more than 6 ounces of fish in a week. It may be especially important for pregnant women to follow these recommendations. Apart from the health considerations, there are very real, very negative effects on oceans ecosystems due to modern, large-scale fishing operations, but this environmental argument is beyond the scope of this discussion. For those working to reverse disease, the best cardiovascular results to date have been achieved with a dietary program that explicitly forbids fish,[27] so that is what I recommend to my patients.

OMEGA-3 FATS (EPA + DHA) AND MERCURY CONTENT OF VARIOUS FISH

	FISH	EPA + DHA, MG/100 G	MERCURY (MCG*/G)
Preferred	Salmon, farmed	2,648	< 0.05
↑	Anchovy	2,055	< 0.05
	Herring, Atlantic	2,014	< 0.05
	Salmon, wild	1,043	< 0.05
	Sardines	982	< 0.05
	Trout	935	0.07
	Tuna (albacore)	862	0.35
	Shark	689	0.99
	Halibut	465	0.25
	Snapper	321	0.19
↓	Cod, Atlantic	158	0.10
Less preferred	Mahimahi	139	0.15

*microgram

Source: Adapted from Mozaffarian D and Rimm EB. Fish intake, contaminants, and human health: Evaluating the risks and the benefits. *JAMA: The Journal of the American Medical Association* 2006;296:1885–1899, which compiled data from numerous sources.

For those who do not consume any fish at all, the omega-3 fat (alpha-linolenic acid, or ALA) that your body can use to make EPA and DHA is present in many different plant foods, including beans and legumes (especially soybeans), green leaves (particularly spinach), and walnuts. You can also consume 1 tablespoon of ground flaxseed or whole chia seeds every day to get lots of ALA.

But here's an important twist to keep in mind: It is believed[29] that the chemical that converts ALA to DHA also works on an omega-6 fatty acid, linoleic acid. When there is lots of omega-6 linoleic acid around (which happens when you eat oils and fatty foods), it may inhibit the process by which ALA is converted into DHA. This is yet another reason to cut down on added oils, which generally have outsize proportions of omega-6 fats.

Vegans have been found to have lower amounts of DHA (a vegan diet does not contain any DHA), but there is no evidence to suggest that this is a problem for vegan adults or for vegan kids.[29] If you choose to eliminate all animal foods from your diet, I recommend consuming 1 tablespoon of ground flaxseed (whole flaxseeds are not digested) every day and eating plenty of legumes and green leafy veggies while avoiding oils. As mentioned above, chia seeds and walnuts also contain relatively high amounts of omega-3 fats.

THE BOTTOM LINE

- The inherent difficulty in assessing the long-term effect of one food group on chronic diseases has created lots of confusion regarding the health effects of consuming fish.

- Many studies have shown improved cardiovascular health in populations eating more fish.

- Omega-3 fats, the prized ingredient in fish, are not the panacea for good health they were earlier thought to be, though they remain essential to the diet.

- Other nutrients and environmental toxins in fish may sabotage health.

- If you consume fish, do so in moderation (3 to 6 ounces per week) and prepare it without added oils or fats. Do not eat more than 6 ounces a week.

- If you do not consume fish, get omega-3 fats from ground flaxseed or whole chia seeds and abundant leafy vegetables and beans. Avoid edible oils, which may impair the body's ability to use omega-3 fats to make EPA and DHA.

Chapter 8

Is Wheat Truly Terrible?

My first encounter involving Ms. Alport (not her real name), a fifty-something woman, was electronic. I received a copy of the lab results that had been ordered by another provider at my office who had seen her for a first visit. The labs were awful—just awful. They showed that Ms. Alport had a terribly low hemoglobin value. Hemoglobin is a critical molecule in our red blood cells that is responsible for carrying oxygen. Hemoglobin can be low when red blood cells leak out of the blood vessels (as with major bleeding after being stabbed in the belly, for example) or if they are destroyed within the blood vessels (as happens in certain autoimmune conditions). Sometimes, the body can just be incapable of making sufficient red blood cells with hemoglobin. Things have to be pretty darn bad for the body to fail at such an elemental, critical function, but that's where Ms. Alport was. Her hemoglobin was about 7. The lower end of the normal range is 11.2. She was profoundly anemic. People with hemoglobin levels this low who are having symptoms (near fainting, chest pain, active bleeding) are given blood immediately. The odd thing with Ms. Alport was that she wasn't having any particular symptoms at all! She was at the clinic for mild musculoskeletal pain and medical paperwork she needed for her housing situation.

She got in right away to get a colonoscopy to see if she had a source of occult (hidden, or microscopic) bleeding in her colon, and the colonoscopy was normal. With further lab testing it became clear she was profoundly iron deficient (iron is required to make hemoglobin-containing red blood cells) as well as folate deficient. She was so iron deficient that it was likely causing her profound anemia. What was going on with this woman who was walking around as if nothing was wrong?

With further testing, we found the root of the problem. She had celiac disease, a devastating reaction to wheat that severely impacted the function of her intestines. She was also diagnosed with osteoporosis, which put her at high risk for fracturing her spine, and severe osteopenia—low bone density—in her hip, giving her a markedly elevated risk for fracturing it, too. Her celiac disease was so bad that she was eating lots of food, but her bowels were just so ravaged from this disease that she wasn't absorbing any nutrients, including iron, folate, or calcium.

All of this from . . . gluten!

After hearing about a patient like this, it is easy to have concerns and questions about the possible dangers of wheat. It seems like a common concern everywhere I look. The popular media are exploding with fear that wheat is the culprit behind many common ailments. From reading some of the books on the bestseller lists, one would think that if we all just went gluten free, we would be slim, healthy, and without disease, like some sort of Paleolithic tribespeople running through the prairies.

I'll explain why I have some very serious concerns about wheat, but I think the blame it's currently taking is excessive. We have gone too far in the battle against wheat, to the point where many are ascribing all of our ills, from diabetes to brain disease to obesity to general malaise, to the consumption of this grass. Too many people are blaming wheat for all their joint aches, fatigue, and abdominal discomfort on the advice of books that then, amazingly, recommend eating unlimited amounts of oils, cheeses, and other animal foods. In other words, it lets them put the blame for how they feel on wheat and continue to feel good about all of their other bad habits.

To begin this discussion, I think it's important to understand how wheat fits into the average American diet. Americans eat a lot of grains. In fact, we eat on average almost 7 ounces of grains a day.[1] To give you an idea of what 7 ounces actually equals, take a look at this list of what 7 ounces of grain is equivalent to.

7 ounces dry pasta, rice, or ready-to-eat cereal	7 slices of bread
	7 small rolls
3½ cups cooked pasta, rice, or cereal	3½ English muffins
7 cups ready-to-eat cereal flakes	3½ bagels

Seven ounces of average intake covers all grains, including both rice and wheat, but Americans consume far more wheat than any other grain, so it's safe to assume that most of the 7 ounces of intake is wheat. And we eat a lot of it. In fact, there are only two food groups that more than 50 percent of Americans get enough of, according to USDA recommendations: grains and protein foods (the protein coming primarily from meat).[2]

Maybe it is true. Maybe we are as addicted to grains as we are to meat. But it isn't that simple. If we look at whole grains, for example, we get a totally different story. We do a miserable job of eating whole grains in this country. Ninety-nine percent of the population eats less than the daily recommended amount of whole grains, which is about 3 ounces, on average.[2] In fact, of all the grains we eat every day, less than 10 percent come in the form of whole grains. So if we eat the equivalent of about 7 slices of bread a day, only about half a slice would be whole grain and the rest would be bread made with white flour.[3]

So, the truth is that we are addicted to *refined* grains that are packaged in highly processed "food mixtures" that contain various oils, processed syrups, and other sugars. What foods am I talking about? The table on the opposite page shows what refined-grain foods we eat and how much of our total refined-grain intake they make up.[4]

When popular books or diet programs talk about people being addicted to wheat, realize that the top three forms of our "addiction" are white bread, cookies and cakes (and other "grain-based desserts"), and pizza. In fact, the vast majority of the wheat we eat in this country comes as a vehicle in multi-ingredient, highly processed food packages formulated to deliver fat, salt, sugar, meat, and/or dairy. One bestselling book[5] lambasting wheat as the cause of so many of our problems characterized America as a "whole grain world."

REFINED-GRAIN FOOD SOURCES AND PERCENTAGE CONTRIBUTION TO OVERALL REFINED-GRAIN INTAKE

Yeast breads	26.4%
Grain-based desserts	9.7%
Pizza	9.2%
Pasta and pasta dishes	7.7%
Mexican mixed dishes	7.5%
Rice and rice mixed dishes	5.3%
Potato/corn/other chips	4.5%
Chicken and chicken mixed dishes	3.9%
Quickbreads	3.6%
Burgers	3.4%
Crackers	3.1%
Ready-to-eat cereals	3.0%
Pretzels	2.0%

Source: Adapted from Bachman JL, Reedy J, Subar AF, and Krebs-Smith SM. Sources of food group intakes among the US population, 2001–2002. *Journal of the American Dietetic Association* 2008;108:804–814.

Nothing could be further from the truth. We are a meat, cheese, and ultra-processed-food world.

When you hear anecdotes about people feeling better after eliminating wheat from their diet, realize that if they started out like the average American, they are eliminating pizza (with all of its dairy, fat, and salt), bread (the vast majority of which is highly refined white bread), cookies and cakes and other high-fat, high-sugar desserts, and pasta (most of which we eat with lots of added fat, cheese, and salt). When you cut these calorie-dense processed foods out of your diet, do you think you might lose weight and feel better? Of course! Is it because you are avoiding wheat or is it because you are avoiding the other components of these ultra-high-calorie processed foods? I'm not sure.

I do not mean to make wheat seem totally blameless. For some people, the adverse effects of wheat consumption are very real. As I described with Ms. Alport, they can be powerful and nasty.

There are three broad categories of bad reactions that might occur from eating wheat. They are allergic reactions, autoimmune reactions, and "other" (neither autoimmune nor allergic).[6] Most people are concerned that they have gluten intolerance without celiac disease. In other words, they believe that gluten makes them feel worse even though they do not have celiac disease. This falls under the category of "other." These categories are not always clearly separated, and like all efforts to define poorly understood medical problems, they are imperfect. Nonetheless, looking at these categories can help you understand what you need to know. What is real and what is overblown?

ALLERGIC REACTIONS

Classically, allergic reactions are bad events that happen soon after ingesting a food allergen—within minutes to hours. Food allergies are more prevalent in young children, and many go away with age.[7] To avoid getting bogged down in the enormous complexities of the immune system, just know that these types of reactions are responded to by a type of antibody called IgE (immunoglobulin E). If your body's immune system is an army, an antibody is one of the foot soldiers with a powerful radio. It engages the enemy and recruits the big-time reinforcements. At the beginning of the process, the food particle, typically a protein, is identified as a foreign element in the body, and the immune system attacks right away in a complex process involving IgE. This is similar to what might happen when you get stung by a bee or take a medication to which you are allergic. The IgE triggers certain cells to release histamine and many other substances (this is why doctors advise people to take antihistamines like diphenhydramine [Benadryl] for mild allergic reactions). These chemicals cause blood vessels to dilate and lead to things like itching, swelling, and redness. People can get swelling of the lips, tongue, and throat, and they can get skin reactions like hives, which are short-lived, itchy, red, puffy patches on diffuse areas of their skin. In severe cases, people can have a life-threatening drop in blood pressure or have a difficult time breathing in a reaction called anaphylaxis. All of these things usually happen within minutes to several hours of eating the food. IgE is a defining feature of this type of allergic reaction because it directs this cascade of events.

However, there are allergic reactions that are not mediated by IgE, and they may take a little longer to appear. These include conditions that cause inflammation in different parts of the gastrointestinal tract (and have fancy names like eosinophilic esophagitis, eosinophilic gastroenteritis, and food protein–induced allergic proctocolitis and enterocolitis[7]). Symptoms of these allergies may include things like vomiting, diarrhea, reflux, blood and mucus in the stool, and abdominal pain (colic). There are also skin reactions that fall under this "non-IgE" category, including eczema, although the relationship between food allergies and eczema is complicated and currently poorly understood.[7]

There are many different foods that have been known to cause allergic reactions. Depending on how you define and confirm the food allergies, there are widely varying reports of how many people suffer from true food allergies. Studies that simply asked people whether or not they have a food allergy found that food allergies are far more common than studies that required objective evidence of an allergy did.[8] Food challenge tests, particularly when subjects don't know if they are getting the possible allergen or not, are considered the best way to test for allergies, but studies using this method are uncommon. The list below shows the food culprits most commonly associated with allergic reactions.

FOODS ASSOCIATED WITH ALLERGIES AND THEIR RELATIVE PREVALENCE OF CAUSING ALLERGIES[7-9]

Cow's milk (the most common food allergen)

Egg (more common)

Shellfish (more common)

Peanuts (more common)

Fish (common)

Tree nuts (common)

Fruits (common)

Wheat (less common)

Soy (less common)

Vegetables and legumes other than peanuts (less common)

Based on recent large reviews,[8] about 12 to 13 percent of people report having a food allergy to any one of the following: cow's milk, egg, shellfish, peanuts, and fish. A smaller number report allergies to the other plant foods on the list.[7-9] Cow's milk is the most common food allergen, with roughly 6 to 7 percent of kids and 1 to 2 percent of adults reporting it.[7] Studies that measured the prevalence of allergies based on actual food challenges have found that only about 3 percent of people are allergic to any of the more common allergens. With most food allergies (excepting allergies to nuts), the majority of people grow out of them by their late teenage years.[7] As stated before, though, none of these specific numbers are very reliable.

Based on these recent reviews,[7-9] wheat is a less common cause of allergic reactions compared to other problematic foods. However, the many studies report widely varying prevalence rates depending on what methods were used to test for an allergy. Reactions connected to wheat have been noted in the skin, gastrointestinal tract, and respiratory system.[6] A small percentage of bakers, who spend all day inhaling wheat flour, develop an allergy to it and have increased respiratory symptoms and runny nose. The proportion of bakers with these symptoms is higher than it is in the rest of the population. Some people have skin reactions (itching and redness) when handling wheat, and, strangely, after eating wheat and then exercising, some people have symptoms ranging from skin itching and redness to a severe systemic reaction (anaphylaxis).

So wheat allergy, while possible, is not something the vast majority of people should be terribly concerned about. In fact, many other types of foods more commonly cause allergic reactions.

AUTOIMMUNE REACTIONS TO WHEAT

The autoimmune reactions to wheat, on the other hand, are serious cause for concern. In this category of reactions are celiac disease, a related skin condition called dermatitis herpetiformis, and a related neurological condition called gluten ataxia.[6] There is also some evidence connecting wheat to type 1 diabetes.

Celiac disease is by far the most prominent and well-known autoimmune reaction to wheat. But what is it? There are many unknown details, but basically a person's immune system becomes sensitized to wheat protein (gluten). The immune system attacks upon seeing gluten that's been absorbed by the intestinal cells. As a result, the small intestine becomes very inflamed and dysfunctional, and this leads to various symptoms and complications. This complete process, yielding symptoms and complications, can happen fairly quickly, over weeks, or take decades. Furthermore, the disease can stall out, meaning that the sensitization to gluten has occurred (and can be confirmed by blood tests), but symptoms never develop. It can occur in infants as soon as wheat is introduced into their diet, or it can appear late in life. A significant percentage of people with the disease are not diagnosed until after the age of 60.[10]

As celiac disease has become more recognized over the past 10 to 15 years, we have learned that it affects more people than originally thought. A 2003 study[11] measured its prevalence based on blood tests and intestinal biopsies and found that of those people who weren't at high risk for celiac disease, about 1 in 133 had celiac disease. Those at high risk include people with a family member with the disease or people who have symptoms or an associated condition. The table below shows the rates of celiac disease among different groups.

PREVALENCE OF CELIAC DISEASE

Among people with first-degree relatives with celiac disease	1 in 22 have the disease
Among people with second-degree relatives with celiac disease	1 in 39 have the disease
Among people with symptoms (chronic diarrhea, abdominal pain, or constipation) or an associated condition (type 1 diabetes, Down syndrome, anemia, arthritis, infertility, osteoporosis, medically diagnosed short stature)	1 in 56 have the disease
General population not in one of the previous categories	1 in 133 have the disease

Source: Fasano A, Berti I, Gerarduzzi T, Not T, et al. Prevalence of celiac disease in at-risk and not-at-risk groups in the United States: A large multicenter study. *Archives of Internal Medicine* 2003;163:286–292.

The most common symptoms are chronic diarrhea, weight loss, and a distended (swollen) belly (40 to 50 percent have these symptoms[12]). However, some people instead have anemia, abdominal discomfort, mouth ulcers, tiredness, easy bruising, liver inflammation, or thinning bones. Some people who have significant celiac disease that is left untreated have osteoporosis, infertility, and recurrent miscarriage. Many of these secondary symptoms are related to poor nutrient absorption once the small intestine is highly inflamed. Other associated conditions are a skin rash (dermatitis herpetiformis) and neurologic complaints (gluten ataxia),[12] discussed later.

Make no mistake—this is a nasty disease! And it all relates to wheat protein. More specifically, it relates to gluten-containing grains, including barley and rye. The good news is that by eliminating the foods that contain gluten, the vast majority of people with this disease can reverse their illness and the bowel can start working well again. If you look at the simplified family tree of common grains in the figure below, you'll see that this one genetic branch is the bad player. Eating small amounts of oats seems to be okay for most patients with celiac disease, but in a few, they can elicit some symptoms.[12] Rice, corn, millet, sorghum (which is not shown in the figure, but is near corn in the grain evolutionary tree) and teff (a grain commonly used in parts of Africa) all are safe for celiac patients to eat, which makes sense because these grains aren't closely related to wheat, barley, and rye.[13]

SIMPLIFIED FAMILY TREE OF COMMON GRAINS

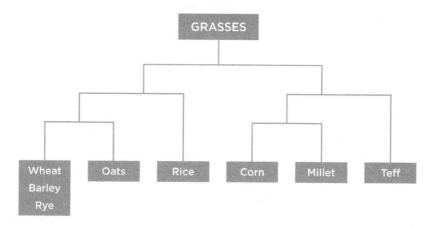

Source: Adapted from Kellogg EA. Evolutionary history of the grasses.
Plant Physiology 2001;125:1198–1205.

If eliminating wheat solves the problem, can we simply say that eating wheat causes this disease? No, we can't, because almost everyone eats wheat and there are about 100 times more people who don't get celiac disease than people who do. So why does this happen to some people? The honest answer at this time is that we don't know. There is a strong genetic component to disease risk. Most people with celiac disease have one of these two genes: HLA-DQ2 or HLA-DQ8. In fact, almost 100 percent of those people with celiac disease have one of them, or part of one of them (most commonly HLA-DQ2).[14] But the genetics are very complicated. There are at least 39 other genes besides the HLA genes that may play a role in genetic predisposition to celiac disease.[15]

But the genes alone are not enough to cause the disease. HLA-DQ2, for example, is present in about 35 percent of all European people and their descendants,[16] and yet only about 1 percent of these people have the disease. Furthermore, not even exposure to wheat is enough to cause the disease. In fact, many people with both the genes and lifelong exposure to wheat are in excellent health until later in life, when the disease emerges. What triggers it in these people is unknown. In other words, the HLA genes and exposure to wheat are necessary but not sufficient on their own to cause celiac disease.

In one particularly interesting study, a group in Finland[17] followed children born with the two HLA genes that put them at risk for getting celiac disease. The researchers measured antibodies in the blood that are associated with the disease. These children were raised on normal, wheat-containing diets. About 4 percent of the kids had positive blood tests that showed they had developed antibodies that attacked gluten-related proteins. You would think that these kids, eating a wheat-containing diet, having the right genes, and having developed an immune response to gluten-related proteins, would go on to develop celiac disease. But in fact, a full 49 percent of these kids eventually spontaneously lost their major antibody to the gluten-related proteins, leaving them without the antibody commonly associated with celiac disease.[17] This happened *while they continue to consume wheat*. Something about the environment, their immune system, or their intestines changed so that they stopped making antibodies to the wheat-related proteins.

Similar results were seen in a French study[18] of 61 adults who had been diagnosed with celiac disease as kids. These 61 patients resumed eating wheat sometime after their diagnosis because they no longer had symptoms when they tried to eat it. The majority of them still had some degree of celiac disease in their intestines even though they didn't have noticeable symptoms. This majority had higher rates of osteopenia and osteoporosis (bone thinning), suggesting that even without symptoms most celiac patients should not go back to a gluten-containing diet. But remarkably, 20 percent of those with a childhood diagnosis were eating a full wheat-containing diet and not having *any* symptoms or signs of intestinal damage or related problems.[18] The researchers didn't know why, but did note that those who were seemingly "cured" of their celiac disease were those who were diagnosed at an earlier age.[18]

Clearly, something beyond just wheat protein and genes is driving celiac disease, but we don't know what it is yet. Viruses may play a role,[19] or breastfeeding in infancy and the timing of food introduction,[20, 21] and there has been interesting work indicating that other nutrients may change the disease process.[22] Studies have shown that variation in the different bacteria that are naturally present in our intestines may also play an important role.[23] But none of this is clear yet, and it probably won't be for quite some time.

Regardless of the uncertainties, we know enough to be worried about celiac disease. It is common enough that every primary care doctor has at least a few patients with it, and it is severe enough to warrant total dietary change. As for Ms. Alport, she went on a strict gluten-free diet. Her bowel habits changed, and she started gaining weight appropriately. With iron and folate supplementation, her hemoglobin and overall blood count returned to normal within about 7 months. As her physician, I was gratified to see her recovery, but it had an asterisk applied to it. She was left with a serious bone density problem at a relatively young age.

This is analogous to my feeling about wheat in general. I do defend it as a source of good nutrition, but I always place an asterisk by it in my mind because I know that rare people do need to strictly avoid gluten or suffer the very serious ravages of celiac disease. For these people, wheat is indeed truly terrible.

THE BOTTOM LINE

- Avoiding gluten is one of the hottest trends in our culture right now.

- Americans eat lots of wheat in the form of highly processed, refined foods.

- There are three categories of wheat problems: allergy, autoimmune disease, and "other" (non-celiac gluten sensitivity).

- True wheat allergies are rare.

- About 1 in 100 people has celiac disease, a very serious autoimmune cause of intestinal dysfunction that can lead to blood, bone, and other systemic problems.

Chapter 9

A Gluten-Free World

I mentioned three other autoimmune conditions linked to wheat proteins: dermatitis herpetiformis, gluten ataxia, and type 1 diabetes. It is worth quickly exploring these illnesses before getting to the most common problem: feeling unwell after eating gluten even though there is no sign of celiac disease, other autoimmune disease, or wheat allergy.

Dermatitis herpetiformis is a skin rash that occurs in people who have celiac disease. It is a blistering, itchy, burning rash that can occur on different parts of the body, but most classically appears on the backs of the elbows, the fronts of the knees, the buttocks, and sometimes on the neck and scalp. It is far more rare than celiac disease itself, showing up in just a couple out of every 10,000 people.[1] This rash is responsive to a gluten-free diet, so those who are diagnosed with it should be tested for celiac disease and adopt a gluten-free diet.[2]

Gluten ataxia is another autoimmune reaction to wheat protein. "Ataxia" is a term that means loss of coordination of muscle movements, and it can take a variety of forms. For example, someone with gait ataxia who is walking might look like they've had too much to drink. It can be a seriously disabling neurologic symptom. Rarely, people will develop spontaneous ataxia without any known cause. It has been found that in these people, a surprisingly high percentage (about 25 percent) also have antibodies to wheat protein.[2] Unfortunately, the wheat protein looks an awful lot like part of a type of cell in the cerebellum, the part of the brain that helps coordinate movement. So the immune system attacks the cerebellar cells as well, potentially causing this condition known as gluten ataxia. People who are unfortunate enough to have this type of neurologic problem should be tested for autoimmune sensitivity to wheat protein[2] and if found to react, they should eat a gluten-free diet. That might prevent further damage, though any significant damage already done to the cerebellum is likely irreversible.

And finally, type 1 diabetes has been linked to celiac disease. Previously known as juvenile diabetes, it is far less common than type 2 diabetes, which is the kind associated with obesity that we hear about in the news all the time. Type 1 diabetes occurs when the immune system attacks the pancreas. This slowly destroys the pancreas's ability to produce insulin, which is needed to manage and use blood glucose throughout the body. Celiac disease has been linked to other autoimmune dysfunction as well,[3] but its association with type 1 diabetes is most well established. Somewhere around 5 percent of the people with type 1 diabetes have celiac disease,[4] significantly more than the roughly 1 percent found in the general population. Some of the research into what is behind both of these conditions suggests that wheat protein might cause or worsen some aspects of type 1 diabetes,[5, 6] but other studies show the opposite, that wheat is protective compared to other foods.[7]

Like celiac disease, there are an awful lot of question marks surrounding type 1 diabetes. Other foods, including cow's milk and soy, also have been linked to type 1 diabetes. Of all the foods studied, cow's milk has the greatest depth and breadth of research showing a possible link,[8, 9] and it is the food most likely to cause type 1 diabetes. So while there is far more research to be done before anything can be said with certainty, I believe that those who suggest that wheat is the main cause of type 1 diabetes are ignoring a much more serious threat: cow's milk.

NON-CELIAC GLUTEN SENSITIVITY

Up to this point in our discussion of wheat, we have seen that true wheat allergy is possible, though quite rare and less likely than many other food allergies. We have also seen that celiac disease is a very serious illness, one with multiple causes in addition to wheat protein, that affects only about 1 percent of the population. There are some serious associated conditions (ataxia, for example), but these are either extremely rare or require much more research before we fully understand their association with wheat. If these problems were all that we needed to worry about, there would be only a very small percentage of people in the United States for whom a gluten-free diet was medically indicated.

Yet gluten-free eating is an exploding trend, with many more people eating gluten-free food than there are people with any of the problems discussed. In the past couple of years, more than 40 percent of all new food products have been labeled with health- and nutrition-related claims.[10] In 2001, none of the top 10 health- and nutrition-related claims for new foods had anything to do with gluten, but in 2010, "gluten free" was the second most common health claim on all new products carrying health claims.[10] Various surveys[10] have found that about 15 percent of all people purchase some gluten-free varieties of food, creating a market that will amount to more than $5 billion by 2015. Unsurprisingly, these same surveys found that only about 1 out of 10 to 20 people purchasing gluten-free varieties of food are buying it to treat celiac disease. Obviously, the autoimmune and allergy problems we've discussed drive only a small portion of this exploding trend.

What is the missing link? What's called "non-celiac gluten sensitivity." Popular books and many resources on the Internet have embraced the concept that even those without celiac disease who are exposed to gluten may suffer many symptoms and diseases ranging from garden-variety fatigue, headaches, and depression to chronic abdominal pain, obesity, type 2 diabetes, rheumatoid arthritis, schizophrenia, heart disease, and other chronic diseases. The emphasis in these messages tends to be that for those consuming a typical American diet, simply removing the gluten while continuing to eat to the same dietary pattern will result in dramatic health improvement. What is the research behind this?

There is enough research now to show that non-celiac gluten sensitivity is real, but many of the wide-ranging gluten-related illness claims have scant published research to back them up. In other words, at this point the exploding interest in gluten-free foods cannot be scientifically justified as relevant to most people's health. Many of my patients with minor medical complaints and an interest in alternative treatments have taken up avoiding wheat, but there is very little evidence that wheat itself is a major problem for most people. Up until a few years ago, scientists were debating whether such a thing as non-celiac gluten sensitivity even existed.

I don't mean to denounce the idea entirely. Non-celiac gluten sensitivity, when it meets strict criteria,[2] is real and can cause troubling symptoms. In order to justify giving this diagnosis, several things must be shown: that the patient does not have a wheat allergy (confirmed with blood and skin tests) and does not have celiac disease (confirmed by blood tests, genetic tests, and/or biopsies of the small intestine), and, most importantly, that symptoms resolve during a blinded trial of a gluten-free diet.[2] This last requirement is the most important, in my opinion. The way it is fulfilled in some research settings is that all the people are put on a gluten-free diet and then given either capsules or baked goods for a period of time. These capsules and baked goods may contain gluten or they may not, and the patient doesn't know this information (this is what being "blinded" means). Then the patients record their symptoms, and if the symptoms truly are linked to gluten exposure, they are deemed to be gluten sensitive. This does away with the placebo effect, which is a fascinating and enormously powerful psychological/emotional phenomenon affecting health and illness throughout the body.

These strict criteria are almost never fulfilled outside of research settings. Unfortunately, medically supervised, blinded testing of a gluten-free diet is not readily available in most communities. Besides, far more people prefer to try a gluten-free diet on their own instead of being poked and prodded by doctors. Further, these three criteria for a proper diagnosis have only recently been established. I have never met a patient with self-described non-celiac wheat sensitivity who has gone through the steps of confirming the problem, even though I have met numerous patients with self-diagnosed non-celiac wheat sensitivity.

There are research settings in which these criteria have been met, however. One group in Italy[11] studied a group of 920 patients diagnosed with irritable bowel syndrome, or IBS. IBS is a disorder defined as abdominal pain or discomfort for 12 weeks over the past year that is relieved by a bowel movement and accompanied by a change in stool form, appearance, or frequency. It is a diagnosis of exclusion, meaning that there are no tests to prove this diagnosis. Instead, it is simply a name that we use for these types of symptoms when we have ruled out other known disorders.

As you might imagine, this is a group of patients that are likely to have a much higher than average probability of food sensitivities and intolerances. These symptoms are similar to known disorders caused by wheat, for example. So the researchers took 920 IBS patients,[11] confirmed that they did not have celiac disease or wheat allergy, and subjected them to a blinded food challenge. All of them went on a diet that excluded wheat, cow's milk, tomato, eggs, chocolate, and any other foods that the patients had found to exacerbate their symptoms. They did this for 4 weeks, and then they were given capsules containing either gluten or a non-gluten lookalike. All the patients had 2 weeks of placebo and 2 weeks of gluten, but nobody knew what order they were getting them in. They recorded their symptoms. It was found that 276 of the original 920 IBS patients (30 percent) had improvement in their symptoms on the elimination diet and a return of symptoms (pain, bloating, change in stool consistency) when taking the gluten capsule. Researchers then put these 276 wheat-sensitive patients through further testing to examine whether they were also sensitive to other foods. They did the same blinded testing method using cow's milk proteins and found that 206 of them were also sensitive to cow's milk proteins. In other words, 75 percent of those who were sensitive to wheat were also sensitive to milk protein. Unfortunately, these researchers did not explore whether IBS patients were sensitive to cow's milk without being sensitive to gluten.

The take-home message from this study[11] is that even among people with chronic digestive symptoms (IBS), only 30 percent were sensitive to gluten, and most of these gluten-sensitive people were sensitive to cow's milk and other foods as well. This is not meant to discount their sensitivity to gluten, but clearly there is something bigger than gluten going on here. Fewer than 1 out of 10 of the original group was found to be sensitive to wheat alone, even though this was a group of people that would have a high likelihood of having wheat sensitivity. Those who had multiple food sensitivities seemed to be somewhat more likely to have a history of allergies, including allergic eczema and asthma, and those with wheat-only sensitivity were more likely to be related to someone with celiac disease.

Another study[12] in Australia confirmed the reality of non-celiac gluten sensitivity when it enrolled 39 patients with IBS. To be accepted into the trial, these patients were required to have tests showing that they did not have celiac disease and they had to have experienced enough worsening of their symptoms with wheat consumption that they had been on a gluten-free diet that controlled their symptoms prior to joining the study. In no way did this group represent an average group of eaters. These were people with chronic digestive symptoms who already had self-reported wheat sensitivity by fairly strict criteria. Five patients dropped out of the study, but the remaining 34 were given muffins and bread for 6 weeks while consuming an otherwise gluten-free diet. Roughly half the group got muffins and bread with gluten, and the other half got muffins and bread without gluten. Subjects didn't know which group they were part of. The group getting the gluten had significantly more symptoms, including pain, bloating, and stool consistency problems. The biggest difference was fatigue, with the gluten group reporting significantly more. This study clearly indicated that non-celiac gluten sensitivity is a real phenomenon.

But how likely are you to have non-celiac gluten sensitivity? In the absence of a family history of celiac disease or associated conditions and in the absence of chronic symptoms, research suggests you are unlikely to have non-celiac gluten sensitivity. One group reports[2] that about 6 percent of all patients seen at a specialized celiac referral center were found to have non-celiac gluten sensitivity. Common sense tells us that this number cannot be generalized to the general population. After all, to be a patient at a celiac referral center, you would probably be at a very high probability of being sensitive to wheat gluten. Those people with non-celiac gluten sensitivity reported diverse symptoms including abdominal pain, skin rash, headache, "foggy mind," fatigue, diarrhea, depression, anemia, numbness, and joint pain.[2]

At another center, the Italian one mentioned earlier, 46 celiac patients were diagnosed in a year. Another 15 patients had gluten sensitivity alone, and 90 had multiple food hypersensitivity.[11] In other words, wheat sensitivity alone was pretty darn uncommon.

All of this suggests that although non-celiac gluten sensitivity is a real condition with a variety of symptoms, it is almost certainly far rarer than the number of people currently jumping on the gluten-free bandwagon suggests. I suspect that many of the people without celiac disease who are currently concerned about being gluten sensitive are probably not gluten sensitive at all. Like many of the gray areas in this book, though, I would not be surprised if I were singing a different tune about non-celiac gluten sensitivity in 10 years. The research[13] suggests some people have problems with wheat beyond that of the autoimmune disease (celiac), but at this point not enough research has been done to pin much blame very definitely on wheat gluten. Further, there has been no good, standardized study to suggest how common non-celiac gluten sensitivity is in the general population. Research that significantly changes our understanding of this condition might be done and published within the next 10 years.

WHAT YOU SHOULD DO

Wheat gluten is currently considered a great evil in our pop nutrition world. But based on current evidence, I believe this is an inaccurate exaggeration.

I also am disturbed by the popular proposal that gluten is so dangerous that if we just get rid of it we can eat creamy, cheesy foods and meats galore and find good health. This ignores a far deeper and broader body of evidence that dairy foods specifically and animal foods in general are much more poorly tolerated than gluten. Other foods are far more convincingly linked to chronic disease.

But I do find myself with serious concerns about wheat. Celiac disease provides the most damning arguments against its consumption. Celiac disease is serious business. I find myself wondering if we were meant to eat wheat, and if wheat were consistent with health, how could it cause such a serious illness for 1 out of 100 people? In addition, we now know that non-celiac gluten sensitivity is real, despite the fact that it may be uncommon. I have made this same argument against dairy, too. If it were healthy to be the only species on earth to consume large quantities of the lactation fluid of another species way beyond our own weaning period, how is it that so many people are lactose intolerant, allergic to dairy products, and that it is linked to higher cholesterol, prostate and other cancers, and autoimmune disease?

I honestly do not know what the research is likely to show over the next 10 years. It may in fact be reasonable to lessen our wheat exposure. For now, I do not recommend that most people go on a gluten-free diet. Doing so is difficult, expensive, and, based on current data, unlikely to be beneficial for all but a small minority of people. Adhering to a whole-food, plant-based diet presents enough challenges in our high-fat, high-sugar, fast-food culture, but a deep, vast array of evidence supports its enormous benefits. Being gluten free adds an additional, significant layer of difficulty in relationships and emotions[14] that most people don't have to cope with. In addition, whole grain wheat provides lots of fiber and protein, is a concentrated source of energy, and provides several different minerals. My final recommendations are as follows.

1. Avoid the common processed foods in which most people get most of the gluten they eat (white bread, pizza, and cookies, cakes, and pastas made with white flours), and eat a varied whole-food, plant-based diet without limiting whole grains, including 100 percent whole wheat products.

2. If you have family members with celiac disease or you are in a high-risk group (those having certain autoimmune

diseases, severe anemia of unknown cause, or osteoporosis) or have other, more general chronic abdominal or digestive symptoms, talk to your doctor about getting tested for celiac disease. Know that the tests we use to check for celiac disease are much more sensitive (able to detect disease) if you are eating a gluten-rich diet at the time of testing.

3. If you have been checked and don't have celiac disease and don't have food allergies, including wheat allergy, but you have chronic related symptoms, find a way to do a medically supervised, blinded trial to see if you truly have gluten sensitivity. This is nearly impossible to do in most communities, but I mention it here as an ideal. I think this is a good idea so you'll know whether or not you should avoid gluten. Depending on what you turn out to be sensitive to, you might save yourself a lot of trouble and money if you can avoid lifelong uncertainty and experimentation with gluten-free diets.

4. For those who feel so compelled, try a gluten-free diet on your own. Gluten is not required for good health, and a 4-week trial of a gluten-free diet is a safe way to see if you feel better. You must avoid *all* gluten, including wheat, barley, rye, and most processed food products unless they are specifically labeled as gluten free. For a definitive self-trial, I would also avoid oats during this time, since some celiac patients have sensitivity to oats as well. Of course, you cannot be sure you aren't experiencing the placebo effect. You also cannot be sure your health isn't more affected by avoiding the other food products that normally come with wheat, or by the fact that you are likely going to be consuming fewer calories overall. As mentioned above, be aware that the tests we use to check for celiac disease are far less reliable if they're done when you have already been on a gluten-free diet. Do not go on a gluten-free diet and then go to your doctor to be tested for celiac disease.

- Other autoimmune reactions to wheat include a specific skin rash and neurologic dysfunction, but they are very rare.

- Non-celiac gluten sensitivity (what most people are concerned they might have) is real, but also is likely to be quite rare.

- Symptoms of this include abdominal discomfort, bloating, fatigue, joint pains, and "foggy brain."

- Sensitivity to wheat is commonly present with sensitivity to other foods, including dairy, which is the most poorly tolerated food of all.

- A whole-food, plant-based diet, without dairy, is indicated for everyone and I recommend including 100 percent whole wheat. However, I do have an open mind about possibly needing to limit wheat as more research comes to light.

- Involve your doctor, get tested, and try a strict gluten-free diet if you must, but it should not be a first step for most people.

Chapter 10

Organic and GMO

It is hard to argue against the idea of organic foods. Who doesn't want their food to be "natural"? As someone who holds a reverence for the intricate symphony of nature, I find something fundamentally disturbing about the way we manipulate our environment with chemicals and genetic modification to increase output, yield, and profit. Our fruits, vegetables, and grains are grown and processed with chemicals with names that we cannot pronounce and with long-term effects that may not be known. Our food animals are given hormones and antibiotics. And for roughly the past 2 decades our plants have been injected with genes to make them resistant to otherwise toxic herbicides and our food animals are now being genetically altered to grow faster and acquire other attributes. This is a far cry from the way food was grown, distributed, and eaten for the past several thousand years. Against this background, the term "organic" stands as a barrier to modern agricultural practices that many believe to be detrimental to our health and our environment.

Let us start with the basics. What does it mean to be "organic"? The table on the opposite page, adapted from the Washington State Department of Agriculture Web site,[1] shows the main requirements for organic certification.

WHAT IT TAKES TO BE "ORGANIC"

For food crops	Use of land that has been 3 years free of prohibited substances (synthetic fertilizers, prohibited pesticides, etc.)
	Use of natural inputs and organic system plans consisting of things like environmentally sound weed, pest, and manure management and crop rotation systems
	No use of genetically modified organisms (GMOs), irradiation, or sewage sludge and restricted use of raw manure
	Use of organic seeds, when possible
For food animals	Implementation of an Organic Livestock Plan, including:
	Animals have access to the outdoors
	No use of antibiotics, growth hormones, slaughter by-products, or GMOs
	Use of 100% organic feed
For food processing	Implementation of an Organic Processing Plan, including:
	No use of GMOs or irradiation
	No contamination of organic foods during processing

Source: Riddle J and McEvoy M. What are the basic requirements for organic certification? Washington State Department of Agriculture, December 20, 2006. http://agr.wa.gov/foodanimal/organic/Certificate/2006/OrganicRequirementsSimplified.pdf.

What does all of this mean for our health? There are three parts to this discussion. The first is whether organic foods have a better nutrient profile and, thus, better effects on health. The second is the possible dangers of consuming pesticide residue. And lastly, what are the health effects of eating GMOs?

Intertwined with the organic movement has been the recent popular local food, or "locavore," movement. Michael Pollan's books, including *The Omnivore's Dilemma,* helped to popularize this notion that back-to-the-earth local farming (in addition to organic) is not only good for the earth, but also good for you. Farmers' markets are promoted and grass-fed beef is marketed as a healthier option. Some groups even suggest that full-fat milk is healthy, perhaps especially if it is raw. If it is directly from a farm to your table it must be healthier, right?

NUTRIENTS

Unfortunately, with regard to nutrients, there are no clear indications that foods from the organic and the farm-to-table movements have a significantly healthier profile. In 2001, the Soil Association, a UK group with a core mission to promote organic farming, published a report investigating the health benefits of organic foods and found that organic foods possibly have a higher mineral content, a higher vitamin C content, and higher phytonutrient content.[2] Phytonutrients include tens of thousands of chemicals found in plants, some of which are antioxidants and anti-inflammatories and have been found to be beneficial for a wide range of illnesses, including cancer. Plants generate these phytonutrients in order to resist disease and pests as they grow. Thus, if a plant artificially grows faster than it otherwise might because of synthetic fertilizers and never encounters the natural attacks of disease and pests due to the heavy use of herbicides and pesticides, then logically chemically grown (conventionally grown) plants do not generate these natural defense chemicals.[3]

A different report, this time a peer-reviewed journal review article,[4] found that organic produce had more vitamin C and higher levels of some minerals, including iron, magnesium, and phosphorus. In addition, organic produce had less protein and less nitrate. Organic advocates herald the lower nitrate content because it is loosely associated with toxicity on a theoretical level; it may potentially undergo reactions in the body to form nitrosamines, which have been found to initiate and promote cancer when given in megadoses in experimental animal models. Another review article[5] in 2003 highlighted the inconsistency of findings and the reasons for those inconsistencies, but offered some support for the notion that organic foods have higher vitamin C levels. In addition, there was again a finding of less protein content in organic produce, though the protein was of a higher "quality" (it had a better balance of essential amino acids).

An organic industry review published in 2008[6] that selectively included data for analysis found again that vitamin C was slightly higher, protein was slightly lower, and nitrates were lower in organically grown produce. In addition, phytonutrient content was reviewed,[6] and it was found that organic foods have higher antioxidant capacity than conventionally grown foods. The report authors found that organic foods contained about 25 percent more of the nutrients reviewed than conventional foods.

So there may be differences according to some papers, but I suggest that there are unlikely to be major nutrient differences worthy of note. Why? More recently we have heard a very different story. Since these earlier reviews, two large, comprehensive, peer-reviewed journal articles have been published, including one in the *American Journal of Clinical Nutrition* in 2009[7] and one in the *Annals of Internal Medicine* in 2012.[8] Both of these reviews evaluated hundreds of studies and found that *there are no nutrient differences between organic and conventionally grown foods that are likely to be of any health significance.*

Most of the data mentioned have involved plant-foods composition. Animal-foods composition, however, is also very important to consider because I have heard many people, especially those in the locavore or farm-to-table movement, contend that their meat is healthier because of how the animal was raised. Reviews published suggest that there are differences in the types of fats found in some organic meats (namely, grass-fed versus grain-fed) and that there may be relatively more antioxidant vitamins in grass-fed versus grain-fed meats.[8, 9] However, the overall nutrient profiles of organic and conventionally raised animal foods are not that different, according to the review in the *Annals of Internal Medicine.*[8]

We are left with two stories: One is provided by the organic industry and soil advocates; the other is in professional biomedical publications. The organic and soil advocates find there to be nutrient differences, and the most publicized recent biomedical publications find there to be no differences that are likely to have any significance for our health. Not being an organic foods and soil research expert myself, this situation might cause me some consternation. But it doesn't. I believe that in the big picture of your personal health choices, this debate is not relevant to the most significant choices you make every day. Why is that? In the chart below I have put some key nutrient contents of four different foods: 100 calories each of grass-fed beef, conventional beef, organic spinach, and conventional spinach. The nutrient contents are from the USDA nutrient database except for the organic spinach, which I calculated based on the conventional spinach values. For the sake of demonstration and argument, I was generous to the organic folks and generated the organic spinach profile based on the largest adjustments I could find, those noted in the organic industry report[6] published in 2008.

**NUTRIENT CONTENTS IN 100 CALORIES
OF SPINACH AND BEEF**

	GRASS-FED, RAW GROUND BEEF	CONVENTIONAL, RAW GROUND BEEF*	CONVENTIONAL SPINACH	ORGANIC SPINACH‡
Protein (g)	10	7.6	9.7	8.7
Total fat (g)	6.6	7.5	1.7	1.7
Carbohydrate (g)	0	0	15.8	15.8
Fiber (g)	0	0	9.6	9.6
Calcium (mg)	6	3	431	431
Iron (mg)	1	0.75	11.8	11.8
Potassium (mg)	150	108	1,897	1,897
Zinc (mg)	2.4	1.6	2.3	2.3
Vitamin C (mg)	0	0	122	146
Vitamin B_{12} (mcg)	1	1	0	0
Vitamin A (IU)	0	0	9,377	8,627
Saturated fatty acids (g)	2.8	3	0.3	0.3
Monounsaturated fatty acids (g)	2.5	3.3	0.04	0.04
Polyunsaturated fatty acids (g)	0.3	0.3	0.7	0.7
Cholesterol (mg)	32	30	0	0

*Conventional ground beef values based on "USDA Commodity, beef, ground, bulk/coarse ground, frozen, raw"

‡Values of certain nutrient differences calculated from conventional values based on

Source: Benbrook C, Zhao X, Yanez J, Davies N, and Andrews P. New evidence confirms the nutritional superiority of plant-based organic foods. Washington, DC: Organic Center, 2008.

In reviewing the nutrient values of the different foods, it should be readily apparent that the differences between beef and spinach, regardless of production practice, dwarf any small differences deriving from how these foods are grown. You can put lipstick on a pig or grass in a cow's mouth, but you still are stuck eating muscle and fat tissue from a pig or a cow. There are only so many ways muscle and fat tissue can be composed. When the antioxidant vitamins are many hundreds to many thousands times more common in spinach, what difference does it really make that grass-fed beef might have twice as many antioxidant vitamins as grain-fed, when both antioxidant values are minute? The choice is not between grain-fed and grass-fed animals for health. The choice for health in this chart is between beef and spinach. The argument for the possible health benefits of consuming animals raised on certain foods is simply a distraction from the true choice of eating animals versus plants.

The health argument surrounding organic and conventional produce nutrients hinges on differences of 25 percent or so, and the micronutrient differences between plant and animal-based foods can be as big as 10,000 to 100,000 percent. I therefore think it is very misleading for some proponents of the locavore, farm-to-table movement to suggest that you can continue to eat lots of animal-based foods and expect better health. I don't care if you buy your grass-fed beef straight from the farmer at the Saturday market and drink the milk raw straight from the cow's teat; if nutrients have anything to do with health and disease, you're still making the wrong choice. If you can buy organic produce instead of conventional, it is possible there may be small nutrient advantages to the organic variety, but the benefits of switching to a plant-based diet will be much larger, even if you can only buy conventionally grown produce.

PESTICIDES

But how does exposure to pesticide residue affect us when we eat nonorganic foods? Pesticides are much more common on conventionally grown food, but despite the regulations prohibiting the application of synthetic pesticides on organic foods, it's likely that some residues make it on. These pesticides sneak in if there are remnant chemicals in the soil from years past, contaminated water, or liquid runoff or airborne drift from nearby fields. There are protections to minimize pesticide residues, but there will always be some percentage of organic foods that have synthetic pesticides and other chemicals. Given this, it is certainly true that organic foods are less likely to have pesticide residues,[8] and when they are present, they are likely to be present in smaller amounts.[10] This translates into significantly less chemical exposure if you eat organic foods. In one study,[11, 12] a group of kids were given conventionally grown foods and then had a trial period of consuming organic foods. Their urine was collected and analyzed and during the days they were eating organic, they excreted less pesticide residue. When they returned to conventional foods, they started peeing pesticides again.

What effect does this have on our health? I don't know, but there have been studies of people who have had higher exposures to pesticides. Farmers who have been exposed to enormous doses of pesticides all at once complain of a variety of symptoms, including nervous system problems (headache and dizziness), nausea, and skin and eye problems.[13] Among the people who presumably have significantly more exposure to these chemicals through their occupations (i.e., farmers), there are inconsistent associations with cancer. Farmers actually have lower rates of cancer overall, though leukemia, lymphoma, multiple myeloma, and several organ cancers occur slightly more often.[14] There are also several studies that show childhood lymphoma, leukemia, and brain cancer are linked to pesticide exposure.[15] It appears that the prenatal time period, during pregnancy, is the most vulnerable time for pesticide exposure.[16] In addition, there are findings that suggest that pesticides are linked to other birth anomalies and poor neurodevelopment, including low IQ, attention deficit/hyperactivity disorder, and autism.[17] In addition, we know from animal studies that different pesticides can cause neurologic problems, cancer, skin and eye problems, and hormone and endocrine disruption at very high levels of exposure. (You can find specific health-related information for every pesticide at www.epa.gov/pesticides.)

Are you scared yet? If you are, let us back up just a little bit. I have set out a long list of scary potential toxicities, but here is the truth of the matter: There is no convincing research that reducing the small exposure to pesticide residues in conventionally grown produce by eating all organic produce leads to improved health outcomes.[18] And while the toxic effects of megadoses that some of these chemicals have demonstrated in animal studies are alarming, it doesn't necessarily follow that consuming minute amounts as residues in the foods we eat will lead to any toxic effects. Many of these chemicals are known to cause cancer when given in massive doses to lab animals. Extrapolating these results to an extremely low dose in a different species (humans) and trying to guess what the effects might be is very difficult. And there is good evidence that other aspects of food may play a more important role in helping our bodies handle the toxic effects of chemicals we all encounter in day-to-day life. In *The China Study,* we detail an extensive series of laboratory experiments at Cornell University that showed that cancer started by a chemical carcinogen can actually be controlled simply by altering nutrient intake.[19, 20]

In light of these possible concerns, regulatory bodies have established upper limits of exposure deemed to be safe for each of these chemicals. Almost all produce is going to contain levels of pesticides below this upper limit, though there is some small percentage (likely 1 to 2 percent) of food products, both organic and nonorganic, that contain residues that exceed it.[8] The bottom line is that it certainly seems reasonable to try to avoid even the small residues of pesticides in conventionally grown food, especially for pregnant women or young children, in whom pesticides may have a stronger effect, but there is no proof to suggest this is necessary. This does not mean pesticides in food are absolutely safe; it could be that the science has not been done because it is too difficult and expensive to do.

One final, important point: Some of the big, bad environmental pollutants and toxins you have probably heard of, like DDT, PCBs, and dioxins, also end up in our food. They are not broken down easily in nature and are stored in fat cells. Thus, they end up accumulating in greater and greater amounts the farther up the food chain you go.[21, 22] So meat, including fish, and dairy foods have far higher levels of these types of toxins than plant foods. The effects of these toxins at low doses are also somewhat uncertain, but the best way to avoid them is simply to eat lower on the food chain by sticking to plants.

The USDA monitors pesticide residues on foods, and the Environmental Working Group has interpreted its data to assemble simple lists of plant foods that are either high or low in pesticide contamination. This excellent list is called EWG's Shopper's Guide to Pesticides in Produce and can be found at www.ewg.org/foodnews.[23] The table on page 108 is based on that list. Consulting it is an easy way to consider which foods may be worth paying extra for to get the organic variety. This list changes annually, so keeping abreast of their updates may be useful.

PRODUCE WITH THE LEAST AND MOST PESTICIDE RESIDUES

MOST PESTICIDES	LEAST PESTICIDES
1. Apples	1. Avocados
2. Strawberries	2. Sweet corn
3. Grapes	3. Pineapples
4. Celery	4. Cabbage
5. Peaches	5. Sweet peas (frozen)
6. Spinach	6. Onions
7. Sweet bell peppers	7. Asparagus
8. Nectarines (imported)	8. Mangoes
9. Cucumbers	9. Papayas
10. Cherry tomatoes	10. Kiwi
11. Snap peas (imported)	11. Eggplant
12. Potatoes	12. Grapefruit
	13. Cantaloupe
	14. Cauliflower
	15. Sweet potatoes

*Note: *Hot peppers and kale may contain pesticides of special concern.*

Source: Environmental Working Group. EWG's 2014 Shopper's Guide to Pesticides in Produce. April 2014. www.ewg.org/foodnews.

GENETICALLY MODIFIED ORGANISMS

And finally, a quick note about genetically modified organisms (GMOs). GMOs are one of the most contentious topics in nutrition and agriculture. On the one side there are industry and biotech advocates, and on the other side are consumers concerned about human and environmental health who don't like GMOs. What is the big deal?

To begin, it is important to note that genetically modified foods have been in the marketplace for about 20 years in the United States. GMO foods are biotechnology products that have had outside genetic material inserted into their DNA to create plants and animals that would otherwise not exist in nature. The United States has traditionally been by far the largest producer of genetically modified crops. The most common GMO crops are corn, soybeans, and cotton, but genetically modified varieties of rice, potatoes, tomatoes, wheat, sugar beets, and squash have been approved, along with other types of food plants. About 90 percent or more of all corn, soybeans, and cotton grown in this country have been genetically modified.[24] Considering how many products have ingredients made from corn and soybeans, it is a near certainty that you have been eating genetically modified ingredients for years.

However, genetically modified animals have met with more resistance in coming to market. There are pigs that have been altered using genetic technology to provide more omega-3 fats and pigs with a different manure composition. Due to general resistance to eating genetically manipulated animals, these piggies have not gone to market (I couldn't resist). As of this writing, the FDA is on the cusp of either granting or denying regulatory approval to a company that has created Atlantic salmon that grow much faster than naturally occurring Atlantic salmon due to the insertion of genes from a different type of salmon.

Why do we have genetically modified foods, anyway? The lovely, idyllic explanation trotted out by industry and biotech advocates is that with genetic manipulation, we can create food products that are resistant to disease and drought, plants that grow better in less favorable environments, and plants that have improved nutrient profiles. With these qualities, the advocates say that these plant crops will relieve worldwide hunger and malnutrition.

Hogwash. These genetically modified plants are engineered to either resist herbicides, so herbicides can be more liberally used, or they are engineered to directly incorporate insecticides. Soybeans, for example, are engineered so that they are immune to the herbicide glyphosate, known as Roundup. Glyphosate kills weeds that compete with crop plants. Now with genetic engineering, soybean plants can grow and thrive even while heavy Roundup applications are being used to kill the weeds. Other plants, like Bt corn, have been engineered to contain an insecticide within the plant itself that kills pest insects if they ingest the plant.

The convenient aspect of herbicide-resistant crops is that when farmers buy the Roundup-ready soybeans, they can more liberally use Roundup. Indeed, the use of glyphosate herbicide has increased dramatically with the adoption of GMOs.[25, 26] Monsanto makes the Roundup-ready soybean, and guess who makes the Roundup herbicide? Monsanto does, of course. Rather than altruistic motivations, GMO manipulations in practice are devised to create profits, whether by selling patented seeds or the required herbicides that go along with the seeds.

Biotech companies' creation of never-before-seen organisms by using blunt genetic manipulation of food organisms has prompted many raging controversies. There are controversies about the impact on human health, the impact on our environment, and the economic impact, particularly on farmers and segments of the population that don't play along with Monsanto. The economic and environmental impacts are far beyond the scope of this brief commentary, but I would like to make a few comments about the impact of GMOs on human health, given that this is a book about diet and health, after all.

The truth is, I don't feel convinced either way about the safety or dangers of genetically modified foods. We've been eating some types of genetically modified foods now for a long time, and as guinea pigs we've fared okay, at least as far as we know. Over the past 15 years we have become sicker, fatter, more diabetic, and developed more allergies and asthma, celiac disease, and autism, but there are explanations for all of these things beyond eating GMO foods. Further, no particular known negative human outcomes have been linked to GMO foods. The truth is that we simply haven't looked for evidence of any safety or harm issues in a robust way. It is stunning to me how paltry the scientific literature is given that this is a many-billion-dollar industry creating the very food that we eat every day. The authors of one recent review of genetically modified foods wrote that there was "surprisingly limited" data on safety or toxicology when they conducted their first review in 2000 and another in 2006.[27] In their review in 2011, they again state that "studies focused on demonstrating the health safety of GM foods remain very limited."[27]

There have been many types of genetically modified plants. In 2007 one group in France[28] examined a bit of experimental data that had actually been gathered by Monsanto. The data had been released to the public by court order. Researchers studied the effect on rats of a corn engineered to contain an artificial insecticide. It was a small study on a small group of rats over just 90 days. Yet the French group found that rats eating the genetically modified corn had weight changes, triglyceride changes, and signs of liver and kidney toxicity.[28] The French group wrote, "With the present data it cannot be concluded that GM corn MON863 is a safe product."[28] The same group also found signs of kidney and liver changes in rats fed a related genetically modified corn.[29]

Did this set off a firestorm of research with groups around the world trying to replicate these findings, expanding the study to include more animals over a longer period of time? Amazingly, *not at all*! The authors of the 2011 review write, "It seems unbelievable that a risk assessment carried out only on forty rats of each sex receiving GM rich diets for 90 days (yielding results often at the limits of significance) has not been repeated and prolonged independently."[27]

In 2012 a review[30] was published by a different group looking ostensibly at long-term animal studies of various genetically modified plant foods, including corn, soybeans, potatoes, triticale, and rice. By that time, GMOs had been on our plates for about 15 years. After all this time, how many studies did they review? They reviewed 12 "long-term" studies (between 90 days' and 2 years' duration) and 12 multigenerational studies in experimental animals. That's 24 studies for a wide range of GMO products. After 15 years of human consumption and many tens of billions of dollars in profits, they only reviewed 24 animal studies, most of them fairly small and not lasting the length of the lifetime of the animal. The researchers concluded that "the studies reviewed present evidence to show that GM plants are nutritionally equivalent to their non-GM counterparts and can be safely used in food and feed."[30]

But this terribly inadequate body of science yet again came into question more recently with another publication from the group in France that actually looked at the effects of Roundup-tolerant corn and Roundup itself over the course of the lifetime of rats and found that rats exposed to the herbicide and the genetically modified corn had higher mortality with more breast cancer in the females, more liver problems in the males, more kidney problems, and more large tumors in the males.[31] This got a lot of press and met with a firestorm of criticism. Regarding the firestorm, the authors noted that "75% of our first criticisms arising within a week, among publishing authors, come from plant biologists, some developing patents on GMOs, even if it was a toxicological paper on mammals, and from Monsanto Company."[32]

So I am left with an uneasy uncertainty about the safety of genetically modified foods. There are many types of GMOs, and I think that it is entirely possible that at least one of them at some point will have adverse long-term health effects on humans. This doesn't mean all GMOs are bad. From a scientific and physiologic perspective each modified plant can be quite different. But any of these results showing toxicity need to be replicated by multiple independent labs, with bigger numbers of animals, over longer time frames.

But that doesn't seem to be happening. One of the reasons for the dismal lack of data is that the makers of these patented seeds have not allowed scientists to conduct or publish research on their "technology." In an absolutely chilling demonstration of control, according to a 2009 *Scientific American* editorial,[33] when anyone buys a genetically modified seed, they are bound by an agreement with the maker of the seed not to use it in any independent research. Further, after publishing the damaging study[31] raising concerns about one type of Monsanto corn, the journal that published it appeared to go out of its way to make amends with industry. Several months later, the journal created a new senior editorial position for a former Monsanto researcher and biotech industry friend.[34] Later, it *retracted* the previously mentioned paper on Roundup and Roundup-tolerant corn despite taking the extraordinary step of reviewing all of the original data and finding no evidence of fraud or misrepresentation of data.

The impression I get is that the industry has hijacked science. The public is left in the dark. In 2010 a survey[35] found that more than 50 percent of Americans have either no understanding or at best a medium understanding of GMOs. Fifteen percent of people believe GMOs are not safe and another 64 percent are unsure of their safety. Yet we have been eating this stuff unknowingly for almost the past 20 years! The industry is so powerful that there has never been any political will to label foods that contain GMOs. Industry knows this is likely to dent profits, which can't be allowed to happen. So despite the fact that a stunning 93 percent of Americans believe that food should be labeled to indicate if it contains genetically engineered products,[35] the government has blatantly and plainly ignored the public will, perhaps in order to protect industry profits.

The bottom line is that I do not know whether GMO foods pose any real risk to humans. Most of them probably do not, but there may be a variety here and there that does. I just don't know, based on the science, and I don't think anyone else knows for sure, either. But this hijacking of science and politics leaves a horrid taste in my mouth. I personally like to avoid genetically modified foods as much as possible, and at this point I would support any patients who wanted to do the same. There have been recent victories in state governments, namely Connecticut, Vermont, and Maine, requiring that GMO products be labeled in food sold in the state, but this fight is long from over. For most of us, the only way to avoid genetically modified foods is to buy organic, which by definition cannot be GMOs.

- Organic foods may have marginally better nutrient profiles than nonorganic foods, but the much bigger, more important health choice is what food you eat in the first place: plant or animal?

- Residues from pesticides and herbicides are more common in nonorganic foods, but are also present in organic foods.

- There is not a convincing body of evidence proving poor health outcomes from chemical pesticide and herbicide residues, but there is indirect evidence of possible harm.

- GMO foods are unnatural but have no proven ill health effects. However, there has been a stunning lack of research into their effects on human health.

- The only way to avoid GMOs is to buy organic, which I encourage.

- Environmental and social/political aspects of organic foods and GMO foods are largely beyond the scope of my commentary, but they represent important facets of these issues.

Chapter 11

Supplement Mania

There are many kinds of supplements. When we talk about nutrition, we often refer to basic vitamins, like vitamin D or B$_{12}$ supplements. But there are many hundreds of different types of supplements for a variety of illnesses. Many of these go beyond the simple and basic nutritional supplements. An example might be *Garcinia cambogia,* a supplement extract from a plant native to Indonesia. It is used for weight loss. It is known to affect the serotonin system and also interacts with other drugs. It has not, to my knowledge, been subjected to clinical trials as is done with any pharmaceutical drug.

I will focus on vitamin supplements in this chapter, but I am struck by the larger supplement industry as well. I have had several patients with different ailments become somewhat distrustful of the medical system for a variety of reasons. Some of these patients end up going to alternative doctors and practitioners, sometimes paying a lot of money out-of-pocket to do so. Sometimes when they return they have a list of supplements to buy that might cost many thousands of dollars. The supplements may even be sold directly by the health care practitioner, which introduces a serious conflict of interest. I am never comfortable with this scenario because I think the use of supplements mimics the same pharmacologic approach to health and disease as prescription drugs, with the additional major disadvantage of being untested, unproven, and unregulated.

Furthermore, financial conflicts of interest can be much more flagrant in the supplement world than those seen in traditional medicine. I make no extra money at the end of the day by giving anyone a prescription for a drug. My university employer, and many others like it, has barred drug company sales visits, lunches, and "free" samples. If anything, writing the prescription may put the prescriber at risk and can trigger a major paperwork hassle that few people appreciate. But yet I prescribe the medicines if I feel they are indicated. So I have always found it odd that those who are distrustful of this system will go to an alternative practitioner and pay cash out-of-pocket, directly to a practitioner who has a major financial stake in prescribing supplements, for products that may never have been subjected to research trials. Yet this is not uncommon.

Supplements are amazingly popular. About half of US adults are taking supplements, most commonly multivitamins, calcium, or omega-3 fatty acids (fish oil).[1] In addition, I frequently get questions about vitamins D and B_{12} from those who follow a strict vegan diet. There are very few supplements that I ever recommend. In fact, I recommend against their routine use for the general population. This is a discussion to have with your doctor, but extensive and expensive supplementation and alternative health care go together all too often, and I worry that ill effects on patients' pocketbooks and possibly even their health are ignored.

OMEGA-3/FISH OIL SUPPLEMENTS

I covered a lot of the background information on fish oil supplements in Chapters 6 and 7. I encourage you to review that material to fully understand my ambivalence for fish oil. There are few supplements as well studied as omega-3 supplements, and few that have caused as much confusion. In general, there has been enormous interest in the possibility of creating the equivalent of a pharmaceutical drug out of omega-3 supplements.

The largest, most promising investigations have focused on omega-3 supplements and cardiovascular disease. Earlier trials testing fish oil supplementation for the secondary prevention of heart disease showed promise, as they led to a decreased risk of cardiovascular events (death, sudden cardiac death, heart attack).[2] But over time, and over the past 5 to 10 years especially, the studies have found less and less favorable results for fish oil supplementation. Two recent reviews combining data from many different randomized controlled trials have found that there is no statistically significant benefit from taking omega-3 supplements for those without heart disease or those with heart disease, though there may be a slight non-statistically-significant trend toward improved health outcomes.[3, 4] The promise of the studies in the 1990s and earliest 2000s certainly has not been supported by recent research.

The search for a use for omega-3 fats has gone way beyond cardiovascular disease. There have been investigations into whether its supplementation improves weight loss,[5] postpartum depression,[6] stress hormone levels in alcoholic men in rehab,[7] and just about everything in between. There has been a notion that omega-3 fats even make you think better, but one recent review showed there is no good evidence to suggest that omega-3 supplements protect against cognitive decline in older adults.[8] None of the myriad investigations for these other issues have shown major breakthrough results for any significant outcome that a patient would actually care about. There are changes in intermediate chemical mediators, like immune system signal chemicals, when omega-3 fats are supplemented, but that does not necessarily translate into any meaningful health outcome.

There is one effect of omega-3 fatty acid supplements that has been proven beyond a doubt, and that is their ability to lower triglycerides. Triglycerides are measured as part of a routine cholesterol panel. They are fats in your bloodstream that are related to other components of cholesterol metabolism and transport. High triglycerides are a known risk factor for heart disease. A review published about 15 years ago found that marine omega-3 supplements lowered triglycerides by about 25 to 30 percent,[9] and other studies have found that very high triglyceride levels can be reduced by about 40 to 45 percent with marine omega-3 supplements.[10–12] Note that these effects are from marine-sourced omega-3 fish oil supplements, not from plant-sourced alpha-linolenic acid (ALA).[9]

So should all people with high triglycerides be on fish oil supplements? No. At this point there is no good evidence that treating high triglycerides alone provides significant benefit.[13] Since the best benefit has been shown with statin therapy to lower LDL cholesterol, the "unhealthy" cholesterol, recommendations in general suggest just treating with a statin rather than aggressively targeting triglycerides. In fact, one recent study found that targeting triglycerides with a fibrate (another type of medication that lowers triglycerides) among people already on a statin does not confer any cardiovascular benefit.[14]

Even though they can make some numbers look better on a lab test, using omega-3 supplements to lower triglycerides just for the sake of lowering triglycerides may not actually lead to better health. As an aside, if your triglycerides are very high (more than 500 milligrams per deciliter [mg/dL]) or severely high (1,000 mg/dL), then these recommendations change because you may have to worry about pancreatitis. At these levels, your physician should start to be more aggressive in trying to lower triglycerides for reasons beyond cardiovascular disease.

I am ambivalent at best about omega-3 supplements. I recommend against fish oil supplements in the general population and even among people with known heart disease or at high risk for heart disease, because the evidence is not impressive enough to definitely recommend taking them—and seems to be getting weaker by the year. The general institutional recommendation, like that from the American Heart Association, for example, is to eat fatty fish at least twice a week, partially because there is a large body of evidence that people in Western countries who eat more omega-3 fats and have more omega-3 fats in their bloodstreams[15] have a lower risk of cardiovascular disease (see Chapter 7 for the discussion of fish). But these studies were done in the context of a Western diet rich in other meats, oils, and omega-6 fats. I'm left asking myself: How did the most significant angiographically documented reversal of heart disease[16] work without any fish at all?

In light of the greater supporting body of heart disease and diet research, I believe a diet of whole plant foods, with no added fat, is unlikely to be improved upon with the addition of fish or fish oil. Because of the ongoing uncertainty in the literature, those people eating a strict plant-only diet can eat a tablespoon of ground flaxseed or chia seed once a day to ensure adequate omega-3 fat intake along with eating plenty of leafy greens and legumes and avoiding added fats to minimize their intake of omega-6 fats (I discussed the importance of the omega-6–to–omega-3 ratio in Chapter 7).

GENERAL MULTIVITAMIN SUPPLEMENTS

My impression has always been that many people view multivitamins as some sort of insurance policy that they use so they'll feel that they've got their bases covered when it comes to nutrition. Unfortunately, it's an insurance policy that won't pay out and in some cases may be harmful, but people have been buying and taking multivitamins since the first one was introduced in the 1940s.[17] I never recommend a multivitamin for general health. I think it's a waste of money, and generally the scientific authorities agree.

A National Institutes of Health State-of-the-Science Panel was convened to examine the issue of vitamin and mineral supplements for the prevention of chronic disease. By "chronic disease," I mean illnesses like cancer and heart, endocrine, musculoskeletal, neurological, and sensory disease, among others. The expert panel found that "the present evidence is insufficient to recommend either for or against the use of multivitamins by the American public to prevent chronic disease."[17] Evidence suggests that multivitamin supplements do not protect against cardiovascular disease.[18] There are conflicting studies on multivitamins' effect on cancer.[19] Some studies have shown some small benefits,[19] while others have actually shown an *increased* risk of cancer, most famously the trials showing higher rates of lung cancer among smokers taking beta-carotene.[20] There have been some studies showing benefits with certain vitamin and zinc formulations for eye health, specifically macular degeneration,[21, 22] but not cataracts.[23]

In general, the story of multivitamins is a perfect example of reductionism in nutrition research. The pattern that continues to repeat is that observational studies (in which scientists simply record and analyze factors and outcomes, without intervention) find that those people with higher intake or higher blood levels of single vitamins have lower rates of certain diseases. Rather than stop there and focus on trying to get everyone to adopt healthier dietary patterns with more of those vitamins, researchers progress to studying whether pills with those isolated vitamins or minerals can have the same beneficial effect. Isolated nutrients will never have the same beneficial effect as healthy whole foods, as has been shown time and time again in repeated failed trials of vitamins. This is covered in greater detail in *The China Study* and in *Whole*.

In addition, multivitamins are not necessarily benign. There is evidence in some studies that risk of certain cancers in some patient groups is increased with supplement use.[17] In addition, there may be a higher risk of kidney stones and heart attacks in those who use calcium supplements. Vitamin and mineral supplements can be a significant cause of poisoning in children,[24] and birth defects and liver damage have been associated with excess vitamin A ingestion.[25] The National Institutes of Health panel wrote, "There is evidence, however, that certain ingredients in [multivitamin/mineral] supplements can produce adverse effects. ... Although these studies are not definitive, they do suggest possible safety concerns that should be monitored for primary components of multivitamins."[17] For all of these reasons, I propose that you avoid a general multivitamin supplement for maintaining overall health.

CALCIUM

The number one reason people take calcium is for bone health.[1] It has been pushed aggressively as part of dairy campaigns and in supplement campaigns. Postmenopausal women, especially, have been urged to take the supplements to avoid osteoporosis. The popular rationale is very simple: Bone requires calcium for growth and maintenance, and if we don't have enough calcium, then these key processes will falter. While there is a kernel of truth to this rationale, it is extremely simplistic. If we thought the same way about our brains, it might be recommended that we all eat as much brain as possible, right? Eat those neurons!

In reality, the bone growth and maintenance processes are extremely complex. They involve hormone systems like your parathyroid hormone system, other macronutrients like protein, many other micronutrients like sodium, vitamins D and K, exercise, and kidney function. The idea that we can just put more calcium in our mouths and have better bones is a wonderful thought, but it ignores a very complex network of processes prior to the calcium actually getting into the bone. In fact the science has now shown that our ridiculously simplistic calcium-related notions don't reflect reality. Much of the research investigates calcium along with vitamin D, because these two nutrients work together in these processes and so they are often supplemented together for bone health.

Authors of a recent review[26] summarize, "We did not find any consistent evidence on the effects of calcium on bone health in premenopausal women or men. Also, the evidence that calcium supplementation reduces fracture incidence is scarce and inconsistent." If you grew up in the United States, this is pretty shocking stuff. Calcium and its benefit for bone health is one of the core teachings in our country.

In fact, the Institute of Medicine has published similar findings in their recent report. The panel writing the report says, "The benefit of vitamin D and calcium on fractures in community-dwelling individuals was inconsistent across trials."[27] There was evidence for fracture reduction among institutionalized patients[27] (nursing home patients, for example), but not among those still living out in the community. These reports aren't isolated anomalies. The US Preventive Services Task Force recently released a report[28] saying the evidence was not sufficient to recommend for or against vitamin D and calcium supplements for premenopausal women or men of any age. For postmenopausal women, they actually recommend *against* lower-dose vitamin D and calcium supplements for community-dwelling healthy women. They recommend *against* because there is no benefit and there may be harms, including an increased risk of kidney stones.[28]

The picture gets even bleaker. A recent review[29] of multiple studies found that calcium supplements may be linked to worse cardiovascular health. Those taking calcium supplements in randomized trials were more likely to have heart attacks, and there was a trend of more strokes and more death. Yikes! Are you getting the picture?

My final recommendation: If you have major risk factors such as being at high risk for falling, you have osteoporosis or previous fractures, or you are institutionalized, discuss calcium supplementation with your doctor; it may be a worthwhile supplement to take. But if you are otherwise healthy and living in the community, regardless of your age or sex, I do not suggest you take calcium supplements, but rather do the lifestyle changes mentioned below.

Those people who avoid all dairy foods (a good idea) but who also avoid consuming lots of vegetables (a bad idea) may be at risk for calcium deficiency. For a strict plant-based diet, I strongly recommend you eat several servings of calcium-rich vegetables daily, especially dark leafy greens like kale. Beans and just about any other whole vegetable will have calcium as well. Similarly, a serving a day of a nondairy beverage enriched with added calcium will ensure that you get plenty. Among those on a strict plant-based diet, there appears to be no increased risk of fracture as long as they consume at least 525 milligrams of calcium a day.[30] In fact, those with plant-rich diets containing adequate calcium have been shown to have a vastly improved risk of fracture.[31] In addition to these dietary changes for bone health, I strongly recommend regular exercise.[32] These natural changes will go much further than a calcium supplement will ever go.

VITAMIN D

Vitamin D is not really even a vitamin in the sense that it is not necessary for us to consume it in our diets. As many health-savvy people already know, our skin makes vitamin D upon exposure to ultraviolet B (UVB) radiation, a component of sunlight. The chemical made in the skin then travels to the liver and then on to the kidney to undergo two reactions that turn it into the active form of vitamin D. Few foods naturally contain vitamin D. Fish liver, mushrooms, certain types of oily fish, and a few other foods contain some vitamin D. Cow's milk has been supplemented with vitamin D for many decades to prevent rickets.

If you have had any exposure to medical nutrition research in the past several years, you know that vitamin D has been all the scientific rage, with many investigations under way to discern its relationship to a wide variety of diseases and ailments. Vitamin D is integrally involved in calcium absorption and bone growth and remodeling, and it has been linked to a reduced risk of certain cancers, multiple sclerosis, frailty, falls, and many other ailments.[33] Yet for all the interest, results have not consistently shown that supplementing with vitamin D in a pill actually does anything useful for chronic diseases.[27] It has been shown in some studies to slightly reduce the risk of falls, especially in deficient people, such as institutionalized older adults.[34]

Getting enough vitamin D from the sun is easy to do in the spring, summer, and fall, no matter how far from the equator you live. Factors that make a difference in how much vitamin D you make include skin color (the darker your skin color, the less you make), time of day, length of day, and skin covering, including sunblock.[33] If you have exposure on the arms and legs to the midday sun (between 10:00 a.m. and 3:00 p.m.) for 5 to 30 minutes twice a week, you will get sufficient vitamin D.[35] For pale skin you might need as little as 5 minutes, and for dark skin you might need at least 30 minutes. You can make vitamin D even on cloudy days. Clouds, shade, and heavy air pollution or smog clouds reduce vitamin D synthesis by about 50 to 60 percent,[33] but you'll still be making it. Windows block UVB radiation (but not all of the "tanning" radiation, UVA), so you won't make any vitamin D driving in a car unless the windows are down. Sunblock of any reasonable SPF stops almost all vitamin D synthesis[36] on the skin to which it is applied.

In the winter it is more difficult to make adequate vitamin D, particularly in areas far from the equator. The body can store vitamin D and release it throughout the winter,[35] but there is no doubt that many people are at risk for deficiency at that time of year, which brings me to the most important question: When do we care about vitamin D?

I never recommend vitamin D supplementation for preventing most chronic disease (because that has never been shown to be effective), but severe vitamin D deficiency does cause rickets and osteomalacia (in children and adults, respectively), both of which are problems with bone mineralization resulting from inadequate calcium and phosphorus. Vitamin D helps with calcium absorption in the intestine. Very low vitamin D causes insufficient calcium absorption, which triggers other changes, including low phosphorus and hormone system changes. Rickets and osteomalacia are uncommon, but they are very real risks for certain populations.

I consider vitamin D a possible problem only at certain times of the year or in certain populations. It is difficult in the winter months for many to get outside and, even if they can get out, to make adequate vitamin D if they are too far from the equator. For those in the northern (or far southern) latitudes with long winters and little outdoor time, I do recommend taking a vitamin D supplement in the winter months, preferably at least 600 IU per day for those ages 9 years and older.

At any time of year, there are some populations I consider to be at high risk for deficiency: institutionalized people (e.g., nursing home residents), women who wear religious coverings over their entire bodies, very obese people, and exclusively breastfed infants, particularly African American infants born in the northern areas in the wintertime. (If everyone were exposed to an equal amount of sun, people with darker skin would make less vitamin D than people with light skin because of skin pigmentation.) What do all of these people have in common? Their skin may never be exposed to UVB radiation. Elderly institutionalized people should get at least 800 IU a day. This is perhaps the most likely population to get additional benefit from vitamin D supplements (beyond avoiding bone problems) in that they may experience a lower risk of falls with supplementation.[34] Women wearing religious coverings completely over their bodies should take at least 600 IU per day year-round.

For the many adults in the categories above who should supplement, taking 1,000 to 2,000 IU per day is a fine starting point. It's important to note that more is not better with vitamin D. Sometimes more is toxic. If you take more than 4,000 IU per day (the upper limit is significantly less than that for babies), you are above the "tolerable upper limit" set by the Institute of Medicine and at risk for toxicity.[27] There is an easy blood test to check vitamin D levels, which you can discuss with your doctor if you have concerns.

Regarding children, the American Academy of Pediatrics has recommended that infants under 6 months avoid all sun exposure 100 percent of the time to lower their risk of skin cancer, so a lot of parents are undoubtedly following this guideline religiously. Unfortunately, this recommendation puts babies at high risk for rickets and bone problems unless they are supplemented with vitamin D. All infant formulas now have added vitamin D, but breast milk, though it may have a little vitamin D depending on the mom's level, will not have enough to prevent deficiency if the infant never has any skin exposed to the sun.

Authors of a study done in Ohio suggest that a baby wearing only a diaper with about 30 minutes of exposure a week and a fully clothed baby without a hat with about 2 hours a week of exposure will get more than enough sun to avoid severe vitamin D deficiencies.[37] The dilemma is that excess sun exposure is a cause of skin cancer, and it is important to note that infants' skin may burn more easily than adults'. Of course, they won't tell you if they are getting burned until it is way, way too late and they are screaming in pain. It is very reasonable to keep babies out of prolonged direct sunlight, but highly unreasonable to obsess over every 1-minute exposure to the outdoor world they may have. In fact, outdoor time can be healthy and enjoyable, as long as reasonable precautions are taken. For those infants who are exclusively breastfed, especially those who have dark skin and live in northern climates, I recommend giving 400 IU daily of vitamin D to prevent rickets.

One final note: Obesity has been found to correlate with lower vitamin D levels.[27] Vitamin D can be stored in fat, and those who have more fat cells may have a deficiency of active vitamin D because what they have is stored in their fatty tissue. This is yet another reason to maintain a healthy weight. Clinically, I am also slightly more concerned about vitamin D deficiency in obese individuals.

VITAMIN B_{12}

B_{12} is made only in nature by bacteria. Some plant-eating animals, the ruminants, absorb B_{12} made by bacteria in their gastrointestinal tracts. Unfortunately, as far as we know, humans do not. The major natural source of B_{12} for humans is animal foods, including meat, milk, and eggs. Fish and shellfish can be rich sources. There are just a couple of plants that contain an active form of B_{12} (very specific types of algae and mushrooms).[38] Plants in general can absorb B_{12} if they are grown in B_{12}-rich soil or water,[38] but you certainly cannot rely only on plants to satisfy your B_{12} requirement.

B_{12} is an essential nutrient. We *must* have it. It is required for the health of the nervous system and for production of blood cells. Thus, a clinically evident B_{12} deficiency is associated with two illnesses: a nervous system illness called subacute combined degeneration of the spinal cord,[39-41] which causes weakness, numbness, pins-and-needles tingling, and nerve dysfunction in the arms and legs, and a type of anemia (megaloblastic anemia) where the body cannot produce sufficient red blood cells. The anemia can lead to fatigue, pallor, and shortness of breath if it becomes advanced. Nervous system changes are often reversible, but sadly are sometimes irreversible.[41, 42] Beyond those classic syndromes, B$_{12}$ deficiency has been linked to vague psychiatric symptoms, including irritability, memory problems, depression, and psychosis.[43-45] There are also complicated links between B$_{12}$ deficiency and worsened cardiovascular health, including problems with blood vessel function[46] and heart-rate regulation.[47] Poor bone health may be associated with low B$_{12}$ as well.[48, 49] Many of these secondary associations are complicated, and frequently they are not resolved simply by increasing B$_{12}$ levels with supplements.[50] Clearly, we have a lot to learn.

This list of potential problems might lead you to expect that growing infants need B$_{12}$, and indeed they do. Infants with B$_{12}$ deficiency can have a serious failure of development.[51] This means that pregnant and breastfeeding women have to make sure they have enough B$_{12}$ themselves.

There are many reasons that people become deficient in B$_{12}$. It cannot be absorbed if they have a dysfunctional intestine (as in those with Crohn's disease or celiac disease, for example) or if they have a dysfunctional stomach (autoimmune pernicious anemia, for example). People who have had major bowel surgery, like bariatric surgery or surgery to remove part of their intestine, can have B$_{12}$ deficiency. In addition, medications can interfere with B$_{12}$ absorption, including the class of very common acid-suppressing heartburn medications like omeprazole (Prilosec), pantoprazole (Protonix), lansoprazole (Prevacid), and esomeprazole (Nexium).[52]

In addition, you can be at risk for becoming deficient in B$_{12}$ if you don't consume it in your diet. Many foods are supplemented with small amounts of B$_{12}$, including nondairy milks and breakfast cereals, but this may not be enough. That is why I recommend that all people who limit or eliminate animal foods from their diets take a daily B$_{12}$ supplement.

The best-absorbed B$_{12}$ supplements are those that are chewable or dissolvable before swallowing, because this allows the key mouth digestion step to occur before the vitamin lands in the stomach. Just swallowing a whole, intact pill like we do for many medications can be dramatically less effective.[53] Healthy kids and adults will do just fine with 100 micrograms of B$_{12}$ a day. There are two forms of B$_{12}$ that you can buy: cyanocobalamin and methylcobalamin. Methylcobalamin is the metabolically active form found naturally in our bodies, but both types have been shown to increase blood levels of B_{12} without adverse effects. I don't care about the form nearly as much as I care about whether someone is taking it or not.

And lastly, those people with deficiencies or who are at risk for deficiencies should consult their doctors. There are simple blood tests to check blood levels, and some people with some of the problems mentioned above may consider with their doctor other doses and other methods, including injections, of B_{12} administration.

As with all vitamins, I recommend just enough supplementation to avoid clinical deficiency. This means that most people should supplement with a large enough dose that they are just in the range of "normal" lab test results. The goal is to avoid acute deficiency, which is when biological processes fail due to a lack of it. I do not believe in taking vitamin supplements for promoting general long-term health or preventing chronic disease.

THE BOTTOM LINE

- Supplements are largely unnecessary and have proven to be ineffective oversimplifications of what we observe in nature.

- Multivitamins are not beneficial for any chronic diseases (with the exception of some specific formulations in people with macular degeneration). Do not take multivitamins.

- Fish oil most recently has been shown to be ineffective for heart disease, stroke, and any other outcome. Do not take fish oil unless prescribed by your doctor, possibly for a very high triglyceride level.

- Calcium supplements show inconsistent evidence of improving bone health (particularly preventing fractures). If you are otherwise healthy and living independently in the community, do not take calcium supplements, but do eat lots of whole-plant foods and exercise regularly.

- Vitamin D can be a problem in areas far north or south of the equator. Take a supplement (1,000 to 2,000 IU) daily if you are at risk for deficiency.

- All people, particularly breastfeeding or pregnant women, who limit animal-food consumption need to take a daily vitamin B_{12} supplement.

Chapter 12

The Art of Feeding ~~Monkeys~~ Children

When I was a kid growing up, I didn't much care about nutrition, health, medicine, or anything related to those topics. Mostly, I just wanted to go work on the tree house, ski, play board games, collect baseball cards, or pursue a variety of other nerdy activities. I had this vague sense that my dad was a successful nutrition researcher, but I cared much more about the "evil" dad who endorsed child labor by forcing me to help spread mulch around the yard on Saturday mornings, and the "evil" dad who unscrewed the TV cable and hid it when he got fed up with us watching TV or playing video games.

When I was in my early teens, my mom slowly started feeding the family a little differently. We stopped eating as much meat. Chicken became something to flavor the rice once in a while. I ate my last hamburger at a highway rest stop—a fast-food hamburger that contained inconsistencies I could no longer ignore, inconsistencies that recalled thick arterial walls and bits of cartilage. We stopped putting cow's milk on our cereal and instead starting using the limited forms of soy milk that were available. They were powdery mixes that took some time to get used to!

We were otherwise pretty normal. There were no long, flowing linen or hemp skirts, no family drum circles or tree spirit prayers, but my friends certainly knew I ate differently than they did. When the bus stopped at a fast-food joint after my away soccer games, I got to be the weirdo ordering something a little different or not ordering at all. I don't recall if my family or I ever used the word "vegetarian" during this early transition, but we were definitely sliding down that slope.

But this was still just a sideshow to my life. I had many more important things to tend to, like improving my hacky sack skills. So when I was at a friend's house and his sister was mulling the incomprehensible prospect of not eating meat and asking me what my family ate, I didn't even know what to say. "I don't know," I said. "Plants?"

Now that I'm older and a doctor, I encounter people who want to change their diets, some to even try cutting out animal foods or processed foods, and one of the key anxieties they have is what to do with their kids. After all, parents can have a very visceral understanding that kids are just rearranged food components, right? Put a bunch of breast milk or formula in for a while, go to the doctor, and see on the chart how they have grown!

Don't they need certain nutrients? Will they get enough calcium? Iron? Protein? Will they grow strong and be smart and have the future you want them to have without eating a "balanced" diet with cow's milk and meat? Pursuing a little dietary experiment on yourself is one thing, but no one wants to do dietary experiments on their children.

Before we get into the details, here is the crux: The dietary pattern that is healthful for you as an adult is also healthful for your kids.

STARTING FROM CONCEPTION

Let us start with pregnancy. It turns out that nutrition during pregnancy may be important for your child's lifelong health outcomes. In 2003, a landmark research study was published in which researchers gave dietary supplements to pregnant mice of a certain breed and found that the fur color of their offspring was different from the fur color of offspring of unsupplemented mothers.[1] Dietary supplementation also prevented obesity from being "passed" from generation to generation in these mice.[2] Pretty dramatic stuff! In other words, although the genetic code remained the same, gene expression was dramatically altered simply by slightly changing nutrient intake, and this in turn affected the lifelong health (and appearance) of the offspring mice. The principle that environmental exposure regulates gene expression has been around for decades, but the field has recently taken off with genetic technology. This burgeoning field is called epigenetics. Evidence suggests that there are key times in development when environmental exposure influences lifelong risks. For example, does our mom's exposure to food or chemicals while we are developing in her uterus help to determine our risk for heart disease or cancer?[3]

This all serves to remind us that, indeed, nutrition matters. Nutrition matters even before a woman gets pregnant. It turns out that starting a pregnancy while being overweight or obese carries greater health risks for both mom and baby. In one study, being obese significantly increased the risks during pregnancy of high blood pressure, preeclampsia (a disorder that can lead to maternal seizures and other poor outcomes), diabetes, Caesarean section, and large babies, and after pregnancy is linked to childhood obesity.[4] Excessive weight gain during pregnancy also may be a risk for some of these bad outcomes, though the evidence for that is weaker.[4, 5]

What is a healthy weight gain during pregnancy? According to a recent Institute of Medicine Report,[5] it depends on your starting body size. Overweight women should gain less weight than underweight women during pregnancy. The table below shows the suggested weight-gain ranges for each body type.

RECOMMENDED WEIGHT GAIN DURING PREGNANCY

PREPREGNANCY BMI (KG/M²)	RECOMMENDED WEIGHT GAIN (LBS)
Underweight (<18.5)	28–40
Normal weight (18.5–24.9)	25–35
Overweight (25–29.9)	15–25
Obese (>30)	11–20

Source: Rasmussen KM and Yaktine AL, eds. *Weight gain during pregnancy: Reexamining the guidelines.* Committee to Reexamine IOM Pregnancy Weight Guidelines. Washington, DC: National Academies Press, 2009.

If we know what reduces the risk of obesity, high blood pressure, and diabetes at other stages of life, doesn't it make sense that the same diet would be healthy during pregnancy? In fact the same whole-food, plant-based diet is healthy throughout pregnancy. Vegetarian diets have been shown to be linked to a lower risk of excessive weight gain during pregnancy, and higher protein intake is linked to more weight gain.[6, 7] Higher intake of heme iron, the type found in animal foods, has been linked to a higher risk of preeclampsia.[8] Higher intake of eggs and also cholesterol (found only in animal foods) have been linked to a higher risk of gestational diabetes (diabetes during pregnancy).[9] Healthy plant-based diets provide more magnesium, and therefore actually lead to fewer leg cramps in the third trimester.[10]

Does all this mean we know with exact certainty what the perfect diet is? Unfortunately not. But certainly a healthy whole-food, plant-based diet is safe and loaded with the beneficial vitamins and nutrients that a growing baby needs. Even a recent position paper from the relatively conservative American Dietetic Association (now the Academy of Nutrition and Dietetics) endorses well-planned vegetarian diets as safe during pregnancy.[11]

Are there nutrients you might miss out on with a purely plant-based approach? The only supplement I strongly recommend is vitamin B_{12}. All people with reduced animal-food consumption should take a B_{12} supplement daily, and this is particularly important for pregnant women. Otherwise, a nutrient-dense, plant-based diet provides all that you need. In fact, I worry much more that expectant mothers who are eating the standard American diet are missing out on nutrients.

For example, you may have heard about the well-established benefits of folic acid for preventing birth defects (spina bifida, in particular).[12] (Folic acid is the synthetic form of the naturally occurring B vitamin folate.) It also is a good illustration of how poor our Western diet has become. The story shouldn't be that folic acid deficiency causes birth defects, it should be that plant-food deficiency causes birth defects! Folate is found almost exclusively in plant foods (exceptions include animal livers and eggs). It is recommended that adults consume 400 micrograms of folate (600 micrograms if you are pregnant) daily. The table on page 130 shows a list of common plant foods and their folate content. Beans are particularly rich in folate. Green vegetables are also good sources, but every plant has folate, including unenriched wheat, oats, potatoes, and other starchy foods. If you eat anything made from enriched flour (bread, many breakfast cereals, and pastas, for example), folate is supplemented artificially. In fact, if you eat a healthy, whole-food, plant-based diet, it is pretty hard to be deficient in folate. Many women actually *over*supplement; a recent study found that more than 1 in 10 supplement with more than the upper limit (1,000 micrograms) of folic acid.[13]

Does this mean I am against folic acid supplements? As a public health policy for the population in general, I am actually in favor of it and regularly prescribe this vitamin for women planning to become pregnant. Unfortunately, many Americans go many days without eating *any* vegetables or beans, and the clear benefit with folic acid supplementation in reducing the risk of birth defects is likely to be worth the unnatural approach. Many are worried about the possible risks of supplementation, and although there are conflicting studies, recent large reviews have found no increased risk of heart disease or cancer with supplementation.[14, 15] Women who are sure to be consuming lots of healthy plant foods will be meeting their folate needs naturally, without supplementation.[16] Be sure to eat *at least* a cup of beans every day and *at least* ½ cup of cooked leafy greens every day, and with all the other plants you should be eating, you'll be more than set.

FOLATE CONTENT OF VARIOUS PLANT FOODS

FOOD	FOLATE (DIETARY FOLATE EQUIVALENTS, MCG)
1 cup prepared frozen edamame	482
1 cup boiled lentils	358
1 cup raw peanuts	350
1 cup boiled pinto beans	294
1 cup cooked turnip greens	170
½ cup boiled asparagus	134
1 cup cooked mustard greens	131
½ cup spinach	115
1 large white potato (flesh and skin)	114
1 cup broccoli, boiled	103
1 cup sweet corn	103
1 cup oats	87

Source: USDA National Nutrient Database for Standard Reference, Release 26.

And finally, you may have heard about the benefits of certain types of fats, particularly the omega-3 fats DHA and EPA. These are present in fish, but not in most plants. DHA and EPA are not considered essential, however, because we synthesize what we need (see Chapter 6). DHA is an important component of both brains and eyes, however, so there has been much discussion about trying to get enough DHA into infants for growth and development. It is a tremendously confusing area of research with conflicting results. In the popular press, the issue is often terribly over-simplified. Just because DHA is present in the brain and eyes doesn't mean that if we stuff more of it in our mouths we will have better brains

and eyes. By that logic, if we eat more bowels we will have stronger digestion and if we eat more lungs we will breathe better. Unfortunately, it
doesn't work that way. There's a lot of complex biology between the mouth
and the brain!

The short of it is that pregnant women who do not eat any meat and
their kids should be absolutely fine. I'm not aware of any widespread incidence of clinical harm arising from fatty acid deficiency from not eating
fish. Consume a tablespoon of ground flaxseed or whole chia seed daily,
which has lots of ALA, the parent fatty acid, and then limit added oils,
which can hamper how well you convert ALA into DHA and EPA.[17,18] If you
eat fish, choose very carefully so that it is both high in omega-3 fats and low
in mercury (see Chapter 7). Mercury is a well-established neurotoxin. You
can also take a DHA/EPA supplement derived from fish oil or from algae. I
don't think this is necessary, though: Recent major reviews[19,20] have shown
no convincing consensus across multiple trials that infants born at full
term or even preterm have improved brain or vision development when
they eat diets supplemented with these fatty acids.

THE BABE IS HERE

Once the baby is out, there is one very clear, evidence-based healthy food
choice, and that is breast milk. The benefits are numerous and will
improve your baby's health over the next couple of months and even perhaps over their entire lifetime. And we are likely to learn about even more
benefits in the future, given the recently established science of epigenetics. Long-term changes in genetic expression may be set during
times of rapid development.

If you could get the benefits of breastfeeding from a pill that was sold
by a drug company, every single mom in America would probably be
bound by law to give their child this pill.

BENEFITS ASSOCIATED WITH BREASTFEEDING[21-23]

Baby may have a significantly lower risk of

- Ear infections
- Asthma
- Eczema
- Gastrointestinal infections
- Hospitalizations for lung infections
- Type 1 diabetes
- Type 2 diabetes

- Leukemia
- Sudden infant death syndrome (SIDS)
- Crohn's disease
- Ulcerative colitis
- Obesity
- Celiac disease
- Low intelligence scores and low teacher's ratings

Mom may have a significantly lower risk of

- Blood loss after delivery
- Type 2 diabetes
- Postpartum depression
- Breast cancer
- Ovarian cancer

Breastfeeding moms need to consume more calories, but the dietary principles we've already discussed don't change. The same foods remain healthy and unhealthy. If anything, eating a healthy diet at this point in life is even more important because during both pregnancy and breastfeeding, the mom may be helping to set lifelong taste preferences for the baby,[24] and we all want our children to eat their vegetables! As I said before, all women consuming a diet with limited animal foods should take a B_{12} supplement.

Babies should get breast milk exclusively until approximately 6 months of age, at which time you can start adding solid foods. Fruits, vegetables, and cereals are good first foods. I think it is reasonable to feed a new food only once every few days to a week so that if there is an allergic reaction you know what is likely causing it. Your baby does not need pureed meat, and certainly do not give your baby any straight cow's milk or cheese. Continue breastfeeding for a minimum of 1 year as you increase the proportion of solid foods in the daily diet.

As the solid foods become a more and more important part of your child's diet, realize that fruits and vegetables have fewer calories per cup of food. This is great for adults trying to stay slim, but your baby needs a lot of energy for the rapid growth they are experiencing. This is important for all parents to recognize: Your baby cannot control when they eat, and the signs that they are hungry are subtle until they are really starving. As they get older, they may get absorbed in exploring and playing and not even show the subtle signs, leaving them hungry for too long before eating. Make sure that you are proactive in getting them enough food from a wide variety of healthy options. High-calorie, easy plant-based options for kids after the age of 1 include full-fat soy milk, avocados, and nuts of all kinds. Beans and whole grains also are more energy dense. Fruits and veggies are extremely healthy, but less energy dense. If you employ a wide variety of foods and maintain attentiveness to feeding, your child will have no problem taking in enough energy, particularly if you continue to breastfeed as your child is developing solid-food schedules and preferences.

When do you stop breastfeeding? There are natural limits, such as when a child stops being interested or when Mom stops being interested, but this often is determined by cultural norms. We do what our families did before us and what our community thinks is normal, rather than what may actually be most natural for our species. The World Health Organization recommends exclusive breastfeeding for 6 months and continuing to supplement with breastfeeding for at least 2 years. One expert suggests, based on a variety of primate comparisons, that humans' natural age of weaning is anywhere from 2½ to 7 years.[25] These ages are obviously far higher than typical in America, but the point is to feel okay about breastfeeding until either child or mom has had enough, even if it's for longer than your family or neighbors did it.

What about women who can't breastfeed? There are only very rare instances when women truly cannot breastfeed (certain chronic viral infections, medication use, previous breast surgery, etc.), and when these are present, try to acquire milk through a local breast milk bank that screens the available milk. Check out the Human Milk Banking Association of North America (www.hmbana.org) and La Leche League International (www.llli.org). Try not to give up because of feeding difficulty in the first few weeks of breastfeeding. Feeding difficulties are not uncommon, but think of how well breastfeeding has worked for millions of years, when there has been no other alternative! Find a lactation consultant. Do whatever you can to establish breastfeeding and make it feasible. After breastfeeding is established, when Mom goes back to work, she should demand to have the time and space (not a bathroom) at work to pump breast milk, as US employers are legally required to provide. It really is one of the more important things you can give your baby. If there is no way to get breast milk for your baby, then discuss formulas with your pediatrician or family doctor.

And what about supplements? All babies who do not consume any animal foods and are at an age when breast milk consumption is being significantly reduced should be supplemented with daily vitamin B_{12}. Find the smallest dose of B_{12} you can (probably 100 micrograms), cut it into a couple of pieces, and finely crush one of those pieces into your baby's food. They require only about 0.5 microgram of B_{12} a day,[26] so giving them just about any small bit of B_{12} from a crushed tablet will be enough. In addition, all exclusively breastfed babies should be supplemented with 400 IU of vitamin D to avoid acute vitamin D deficiency, which causes rickets, an acute bone disorder. Vitamin D is made by the body upon exposure to sunlight, and many babies, particularly those in locations far from the equator, may not get enough sunlight. Vitamin D is not adequately present in breast milk, so the vitamin D recommendation is made for all exclusively breastfed babies, regardless of Mom's diet (see Chapter 11).

EARLY CHILDHOOD AND BEYOND

I see a lot of parents with overweight kids who are just totally exasperated that they cannot change their kids' eating habits. "They don't eat vegetables," they say. Or perhaps "They eat junk too late at night." Some of these children are heading straight for a lifetime of serious health problems, and starting sooner rather than later, but the family either thinks nothing can be done or, worse, that being obese is just natural due to family history. Kids have strong willpower, and one of the few things they can control is what they swallow. Probably the parents' battles over food have been fought and lost many times and the parents reached a point where they just gave in.

In many of these cases, I see that the parents are struggling with weight themselves. I think that the most important factor in determining a child's eating habits and health behaviors is likely what the parents' eating habits and health behaviors are. The most important thing you can do for your child is to eat a healthy diet yourself. Try to avoid fighting over food, which is easier said than done, I know. Here are some tips for getting some buy-in from your children.

1. Eat a healthy diet yourself. *Both* parents, if involved, have to commit.

2. Eat a healthy diet yourself. Discuss the rationale for eating healthy with your kids. They are smart!

3. Eat a healthy diet yourself. Get the picture?

4. Be sure to give young children and toddlers frequent exposure to healthy foods even if they don't like it at first. Just because they make the yucky face the first time they have spinach doesn't mean that spinach should be retired! Offer and have them taste it often.

5. Limit unhealthy foods in the house. There should not be any processed snack foods, sodas, or candies anywhere in the house. You buy the food, after all. As nutritional "gatekeeper" for the household, you do most of the food purchasing and preparing, and you control directly or indirectly 72 percent of what your child eats both inside and outside of the home.[27] You cannot get too upset if your kid is just eating what you're buying and putting in front of them. What does "in front of them" mean? It means anywhere in the house when you are talking about hungry kids and salt, sugar, and fat.

6. Keep healthy snacks plentiful, convenient, and available. Fresh, whole fruits and vegetables are available year-round. Carrots, celery, homemade hummus, whole grain toast, and low-sugar jam are some foods you might stock. Put them where they are easily seen and reached (at eye level in the front part of the fridge or in a bowl on the table, for example).

7. Give your child a choice over what foods they want to eat, but limit the choices to healthy options. For example, they can have veggie lasagna (loaded with spinach, tomatoes, and other veggies, but without cheese) or minestrone veggie soup with whole grain pasta. Let them help prepare the food, if they want to. Help them feel in control of the process and you'll get more buy-in.

8. For school-age kids, make firm, fair, consistent, and clear rules about eating. For example, no dessert until at least a good effort has been made to eat the healthy food. Repeating food and taste exposures early on, even if they are unpleasant at first, will eventually change their preferences. There doesn't need to be any arguing over these

rules. If your child doesn't meet your requirements, then dinner is over and there's no dessert, period. It's the child's choice, really, and you don't need to fight over it.

I had a mentor who used this type of rule with his school-age kids, and he recommended it to all his patients. His rule was that his kids had to eat the vegetables or they couldn't have any other foods. If they didn't eat the vegetables, he put their plates in the fridge. The meal was over, and there wasn't any haggling or fighting. It was the kids' choice to make. If they got hungry later, they had to eat the vegetables from the plate in the fridge, reheated if they wanted. I have a feeling that with just a couple of extended battles the kids stopped testing the limits, and they certainly didn't go hungry. They just knew what they had to do.

Whether you use this technique or another, I recommend that you make the rules fair, clear, and consistent *every time,* and your kids will flourish.

This is hard work, and I do not mean to suggest otherwise! But encouraging healthy behaviors is well worth the effort. Once expectations are clear and patterns are established, your kids will more often become partners rather than adversaries. Raising healthy kids will become much easier.

As far as foods go, focus on offering a wide variety of whole grains, beans, fruits, vegetables, and nuts. This is the most nutrient-dense diet you can offer. If they aren't getting daily dark-green leafy vegetables, you can always use calcium-fortified nondairy milks to make sure they are getting enough calcium. Supplements are the same as always—just B_{12} if there is significantly reduced animal food in the diet, particularly if you don't eat a lot of fortified foods like breakfast cereals or nondairy milks.

Do these things and you'll be giving your child the very best odds at having a long lifetime of health and success. This is one of the greatest gifts you can give, and one of the most important.

As the uncle of seven nieces and nephews raised on plant-based diets, I can personally attest that both exceptional physical ability and mental acuity are possible on plant-based diets. We are what we eat, and if you put the most exceptional fuel in your kids, they can truly thrive.

──── THE BOTTOM LINE ────

- Recent research shows that good nutrition is crucial during pregnancy and early childhood.

- A whole-food, plant-based diet is healthy during pregnancy. Supplement with vitamin B_{12} if there is reduced animal-food consumption.

- During pregnancy, consume omega-3 fats by eating 1 tablespoon of ground flaxseed or whole chia seeds daily. Omega-3 utilization in the body can be improved by avoiding added oils.

- Breast milk is far and away the healthiest choice for all babies and has many short- and long-term benefits. Vitamin D supplementation is recommended for exclusively breastfed babies.

- A whole-food, plant-based diet is healthful for infants and children, but a B_{12} supplement remains important. If there is any concern about growth or not getting enough calories (which is rare), emphasize calorie-dense plant foods.

- Modeling healthy eating and living for your children is important. Many strategies can be used to encourage healthy eating in young kids. It is one of the most important aspects of parenting, because childhood is when their lifelong taste preferences and health will be set.

Part 3

THE 2-WEEK CAMPBELL PLAN

Chapter 13

The Campbell Plan: Out with the Old

So you're sitting there saying, "I got it! I want to do it! The benefits of a whole-food, plant-based diet are going to outweigh any difficulties that might arise! Give me the shopping list already!" Well, not so fast. When you're thinking of radically revising something as significant as your daily eating habits, it's worth taking stock of your head and heart before jumping into the kitchen. You're going to be dumping a lot of your daily habits at the curb, and there's a lot more to successfully changing your behavior than a shopping list, so let's think about your mental approach to it all. According to a popular theory, there are five stages to behavior change.

Precontemplation is when you don't even recognize that there is a problem with your behavior. "I'm 5 foot 9 and weigh 230 pounds? Big deal! Everyone in my family is big-boned!"

Contemplation is when you know there's a problem and intend to address it, but have made no serious commitment to near-term plans. "I know I have to stop smoking and have considered a few techniques, but I don't want to set a quit date yet."

Preparation is having a commitment to changing within the next month or so and taking small steps toward your change. "I'm going to change my diet in 2 weeks and I want to make a menu plan now."

Action is actually making the change. "I'm on day 2 of the 2-week Campbell Plan trial."

Maintenance is several months after you've successfully made the change and are trying to prevent relapse and maintain the new behavior. "I quit smoking a year ago, but occasionally I still crave a cigarette."

To assess where you are in the process of change, ask yourself the following questions.[1]

Am I seriously intending to change my diet and lifestyle in the next 6 months?

If no, then you are in **precontemplation**.

If yes: Am I seriously intending to change within the next month?

If no, then you are in **contemplation**.

If yes: Am I currently actively changing my behavior?

If no, then you are in **preparation**.

If yes: Did I change my behavior several months ago and am I now focusing on maintaining my change and preventing relapse?

If no, then you are in **action**.

If yes, then you are in **maintenance**.

Part 3 of this book is for the people who are mostly in the preparation, action, and maintenance stages, but it will be of interest to those in contemplation as well. At the very least, the contemplators will get some confidence that this is doable, even if they still don't want to commit to a whole-food, plant-based diet.

THE HEAD AND THE HEART

I want to consider the factors that will predispose you to the greatest likelihood of succeeding in your behavior change.[2] This is the same list that was presented in the Introduction, but this time I have checked off the items you should already have changed. We will be covering the rest shortly. This is the scorecard recording where you are regarding the factors that will help you succeed.

So, how do you stack up? Is your scorecard the same as what I've shown? If so, you're all set. You're going to fly through this. But I'm guessing the majority of you are not able to check off every box. If so, that's okay, but you have some preparation to do before you really get into the 2-week plan in order to maximize your chances of success.

Factors 1 through 4, in my opinion, are at least partly about getting

FACTORS PREDICTING SUCCESS IN CHANGING BEHAVIOR

1.	You have clear, *personal* reasons that justify a *strong desire* to change the foods you eat.	☑
2.	You have *minimized obstacles* (environmental, cognitive, physical) to adopting a new dietary pattern.	☐
3.	You have the necessary *skills* and *confidence* to implement this new lifestyle.	☐
4.	You feel *positive* about your new dietary goals and believe they will be *beneficial*.	☑
5.	Your dietary goals are consistent with your *self-image* and *social norms*.	☑
6.	You have *support* and *encouragement* from people you value and a *community* that supports your dietary changes.	☑

Source: Whitlock EP, Orleans CT, Pender N, and Allan J. Evaluating primary care behavioral counseling interventions: An evidence-based approach. *American Journal of Preventive Medicine* 2002;22:267–284.

your head adequately prepared. These factors are about having the specific knowledge to justify your choices and desires, and then to implement a plan. Factors 2 and 3 are about practical skills that will be discussed later in this book. If you find that you are unaware of how diet relates to your health goals, you certainly won't be able to check off 1 and 4. If you find yourself in this position, you might improve your chance for success by seeking out further information. Read *The China Study* or take an eCornell online course from the nonprofit T. Colin Campbell Center for Nutrition Studies (nutritionstudies.org). Get the information you need to be confident that changing your dietary strategy will be positive and worth the effort.

Factors 1 and 4 through 6 at least partly involve getting your heart in the right place. You can only check off factor 1 if you have personal reasons for your change. Do you know what these are? I've asked you earlier in the book to think about this question, but it is worth revisiting. If you don't have strong personal reasons, changing your diet will be exponentially more difficult. Getting a $400 bonus from your employer for doing a lifestyle program may give you a little boost of motivation, but it isn't nearly as powerful as, for example, having a personal wish to be healthier for your spouse, kids, and grandkids because of how much you enjoy your time with them. Your heart has to be interested in moving to a better place, which also translates into having positive feelings for the upcoming challenge (factor 4).

Finally, you have to be among a supportive group of people who are going to encourage your change (factor 6). Are you in a relationship with someone who will support this dietary experiment? Or is it the opposite? Do you have friends that criticize your attempts to do something unusual? This affects your heart by making you feel either isolated or connected to those around you. Success will be much easier to achieve and you will be happier if eating a healthy diet allows you to feel more connected. This is like an alcoholic or drug addict needing to reevaluate friendships with those who consistently tempt them to relapse. Do you need to reconsider whom you choose to have around you, or at least reevaluate the way you communicate with them? This will also affect factor 5. If you find yourself reevaluating your social and family interactions based on an appreciation for who supports you, you also may be engaged in the process of redefining what is "normal." Is it "normal" and expected that you will be overweight and eat doughnuts and hamburgers every day? Is it "normal" for all the office staff to be overweight and eat pizza with extra cheese and sausage for lunch? Do you or your friends think plant-based eating entails being a hippie-dippie flake? If so, it's time to reconsider these social assumptions and the way you talk about them with the people in your life as you think about adopting a healthier lifestyle.

I can't tell you how to unravel all of these factors because they are going to be different for every reader. We will review some strategies for navigating social situations in Chapter 16. I do sincerely hope that drawing attention to these factors helps you realize that whether or not we change our habits and behaviors involves a whole lot more than just having a better shopping list. This particular behavior change—improving your diet and eating a more optimal whole-food, plant-based diet—is so integral to your current and future health and vitality. It is very personal. This important journey will be affected strongly by your relationships and this journey will, in turn, strongly affect your relationships. Does your head have the right knowledge to understand why you're doing this? And, even more importantly, is your heart comfortable with the prospect of this change? Is this a change that will be leading you toward having stronger connections with the people you care about? Is it possible that there will be more love in your life as you take better care of yourself? Is there any way for you to optimize these factors prior to adopting a whole-food, plant-based diet?

If you don't have the scorecard checked off in an optimal way yet, spend some time trying to optimize whatever you might be missing. Start to strategize about how to check off the remaining factors. They are fundamentally important to whether you can change your behavior, be healthy, and ultimately, be as happy as you would like to be.

YOUR TIMELINE

As I mentioned earlier, my family transitioned to a whole-food, plant-based diet over the course of many years. We took baby steps. I think my parents transitioned our family first because of a belief that vegetables were probably even more important than we had previously realized and red meat wasn't as healthy as previously thought. We ate more lean meats, fish, and more vegetables for a few years. The research results percolated even more into our lives, and we began avoiding lean meats except as flavoring for fried rice and casseroles. We had more vegetarian meals, but still ate plenty of cheese and processed foods. Years into that, we cut out some of the processed foods and the last bit of the meat. By the time I was done with college I was just a plain vegetarian. I ate lots of cheese, still had a lot of processed foods, and didn't really care about oils and added fats. Then a few years later, while coauthoring *The China Study,* I finally got into eating a whole-food, plant-based diet. The dairy and most of the refined grains and oils went away. That was probably about 10 years after my family had started to make significant changes to my diet.

Ten years. That is a long time, and I continue to work to improve my diet!

It is with this in mind that I tell all of my patients: The information in *The China Study* and *The Campbell Plan* is offered to define and help you understand what I believe to be the healthiest way to eat. *What you want to do with it is totally up to you. You are in control.* There shouldn't be any judgment in your life about whether you are following the plan perfectly or not. Even though I am offering a 2-week starter menu plan to sample the food and various cookbooks, a whole-food, plant-based diet is not a short-term weight-loss jolt designed to make you look good in time for summer swimsuits (although it can be used that way). This is about transitioning to a new, healthy lifestyle that lasts forever. Your timeline for achieving it is up to you.

It's not all puppy dogs and rainbows, though. Along with your control comes a caveat: If you have particular health problems or health goals (for example, if you want to reverse your heart disease or you want to get off your blood pressure pills by losing weight), the benefits you'll get will be proportionate to how strictly you follow the principles of the diet. You may need to make significant changes before you begin to get major benefits. One vegetarian meal a week may be fine for those expanding their taste preferences, but your heart disease or other diet-related health problem will likely continue to get worse unless you truly eat differently and follow a whole-food, plant-based diet strictly day in and day out.

Similarly, there is no way for you to truly assess your difficulties with or the benefits of the diet if you don't try it "all the way." Remember, addiction to certain foods is real, and for some, making partial changes may not be enough to change food preference. It is for this reason that I do suggest you go all the way, cold turkey, for *at least* 2 to 4 weeks as an experiment so you'll have the best chance at experiencing the benefits. Giving it a longer period of time is even better because as you get comfortable eating this way, the challenges of change will melt away and you'll experience many more benefits. The health benefits are the best source of motivation you will encounter as you do the hard work to improve your lifestyle.

You are in full control, but keep in mind that you cannot take shortcuts if you want the best for your health, particularly if you want the best *right now*. If you're okay with getting lesser benefits from smaller changes for any of a variety of reasons, that's okay, too, as long as you are informed about your decision.

Preparation: Optimizing your environment

We've talked about the general mental approach to beginning a whole-food, plant-based diet. Let's get more specific and talk about how you can optimize your environment to minimize obstacles to changing your lifestyle. This is all about factor 2 on the scorecard set out earlier in the chapter: minimizing obstacles (environmental, cognitive, and physical) to adopting a new dietary pattern. We are strongly influenced by subtle environmental cues. According to Brian Wansink, PhD, one of the country's leading researchers on environmental influences on eating and food psychology, we make more than 200 food decisions a day, and we are not aware of 90 percent of those decisions.[3]

In a study[4] of office workers and candy consumption, Dr. Wansink and colleagues measured how many chocolate kisses workers ate under different scenarios. The kisses were either on their desk in a visible location, in a desk drawer and thus not visible, or visible on a shelf about 6 feet away.

The position that led to the fewest candies being eaten was having the visible jar on the shelf. If the worker had to get up and walk to the jar, they consumed far fewer—3 a day. They consumed almost three times more (8.6 a day) when the candy was visible and within reach. Having it out of sight but within reach got an intermediate result (5.7 kisses).[4] The lesson you can take from this simple experiment is to make it inconvenient to get bad food and you'll do much better without even thinking about it.

On the flip side, in Dr. Wansink's study of kids in schools, when the fruits were taken out of a dingy, dark section of the lunch line and put in an attractive bowl in a well-lit part of the line, sales of fruit doubled for the semester.[4] Similarly, foods that have exciting names ("torpedo burritos," for example) were better received by kids than the same foods with boring names ("vegetable rolls").[3] And finally, we are attracted to what seems like the prevailing norm. Kids were much more likely to choose white milk over chocolate milk when the cooler had 50 percent white milk than when it had only 10 percent white milk.[3] All of this research from Dr. Wansink, author of the book *Slim by Design,* suggests that how we structure our homes and living spaces has enormous impact on what and how much we eat, probably much more impact than we might have guessed.[5]

There are two components to eating behavior: food choice and food volume. You probably have heard, as I have, endless strategies to help you eat less. These are interesting and potentially valuable techniques, but I'm going to suggest that your primary strategy ought to be optimizing your food choices. If you choose whole, plant-based foods, you will not need to worry about limiting the food volume. You cannot overeat sweet potatoes and broccoli or brown rice and beans. There is too much fiber, too much bulk, and your body will tell you to stop long before you need to consciously restrain yourself.

How do you optimize your chances of making the best food choices? We can apply the same principles Dr. Wansink demonstrated with the children's food choice: Make the best choices the most convenient, attractive, and commonplace and make the worst choices inconvenient and hidden. The overall goal here is to have to use your willpower as little as possible. **Willpower is fragile and limited, but mindless habits are forever.**

The changes you are about to make will be more successful if you integrate them into your life so they become mindless habits as quickly as possible. The first step is to tackle the demons in your kitchen. However you choose to do it, eliminate the foods on the list on page 148 from your house in preparation for your dietary experiment. Some people are reluctant to throw food out because of the money they spent on it. I hear the same argument for cigarettes. That is fine. If you want to slowly eat your way out of your bad foods, you can do that. Just don't replenish them. Some of the foods I'm suggesting you eliminate are staple items that last for a long time, though, and I strongly suggest you throw those out or give them away. Do you really want something in your house that will demand your willpower to avoid day in and day out? Trust me—it's not a successful strategy. Remember, the goal is to make eating healthy food as mindless as possible.

How do you go about this? Schedule a weekend day for working on a kitchen makeover. Have a big, healthy meal before starting so you aren't challenged by hunger as you go about it. Then go through all of your cabinets and your refrigerator and freezer and haul out the bad foods. DON'T DESPAIR—you'll put convenient, healthy, and tasty foods in the empty spaces.

Looking through that list, do you think you'll have to eliminate all the foods in your kitchen? If so, I repeat, Don't despair! This is the first step in your journey: taking stock of the foods that are damaging your body and making them far less convenient, attractive, and commonplace. In the next chapter, we'll fill up all these empty spaces that now exist in your kitchen and you'll see that you aren't going to starve or have to eat cardboard. In fact, there's a wide range of easy, tasty foods you'll start enjoying. Once you get the hang of it, it will not be difficult; it's just *different*. It's like walking into a room where you've changed the type of lighting. At first it seems a bit strange, but you'll adapt very quickly because of the great foods you'll get to enjoy.

Preparation: The medical and monitoring change

I recommend that as you prepare to make this dietary change, you involve your physician, particularly if you take medication that could be affected by diet. You absolutely must involve your doctor if you have diabetes and are on insulin or oral medications that can drop your blood sugar. Within 1 to 2 weeks, your dosage for these medications might change, and if your doctor isn't involved to adjust them appropriately, it can be dangerous. Similarly, you might find you need to reduce or eliminate your blood pressure pills as you lose weight. Other medications that

FOODS TO ELIMINATE

Pure fats	Liquid oil of ALL varieties
	Butter
	Margarine
	Butter substitutes, including the confusingly labeled "healthy" varieties like Smart Balance
Mayonnaise	
Salad dressings with the word "oil" anywhere in the ingredient list	
Refined grain ("white") flours	"All-purpose" and "unbleached" flours
Refined grain pastas	Everything that doesn't explicitly say it is made with 100% whole grains
Refined grain breads	Everything that doesn't explicitly say it is made with 100% whole grains
Croutons	
Packaged sugary foods	Candy
	Cookies
	Cakes
	Frozen desserts
Energy bars	Unless they contain only whole-food ingredients
Breakfast cereals	All that aren't made with whole grains and don't contain minimal or zero added sugar
	Anything with more than 6 g sugar or more than 15% of its calories from fat per serving
White rice	
Artificial sweeteners	
Cake and cookie mixes	
Hot chocolate and sweetened drink mixes	
Coffee creamer	
Cow's milk	
Cheeses	All types
Yogurt from cow's milk	Yes, even that Greek yogurt
Sour cream	
Meats	Beef, pork, chicken, turkey, and all other meats
Many frozen meals	Everything that contains meat, cheese, or oils
Many sauce blends	Everything with more than 10% of its calories from fat
Tomato sauces	Everything with more than 10% of its calories from fat

can be affected by your diet include blood thinners like warfarin (also known as Coumadin). If you're on this medication, have your blood level checked more frequently for a while if you're dramatically changing your diet. Similarly, you might be able to reduce or eliminate other medications you take for heartburn (GERD), high cholesterol, gout, arthritis, pain, and even autoimmune medications, but all of these changes need to be discussed with your physician.

When you allow your body to heal itself, the disease processes you have been enduring may be dramatically improved, and the medications you take may need adjustment. Involve your doctor.

There's another reason for seeing your doctor, and that is to enable you to monitor your body's reaction to your dietary shift. There are many ways to monitor any lifestyle change, including:

1. Recording food intake

2. Recording energy output
   (exercise, number of steps taken, etc.)

3. Recording health outcomes

When we monitor our efforts, we tend to be more effective. When we are conscious of what foods we eat, we are aware of any lapses we have and do a better job of avoiding them. In the National Weight Control Registry, a registry of individuals who have successfully lost weight and maintained the loss, people who stopped weighing themselves frequently regained more weight.[6]

If you are interested in weight loss, I suggest you try recording your food intake, at least for a short time. You can do this with varying amounts of effort, but chances are that the more you stay aware of what you eat, the more weight you will lose. There are now a variety of smartphone applications that allow you to input your recipes and foods, and even scan bar codes and then automatically calculate your calorie intake. Keeping a food diary, particularly if you use a fancy app that calculates your nutrient intake, can be useful not only for those who want to lose weight, but also for those of us who are curious about the nutrients we consume. This method of monitoring your food intake can increase your confidence that you are in fact doing great things for yourself (factor 3 on the scorecard).

I also recommend that you record how your health improves. There are a couple of ways to do this that are easy, cheap, and convenient. One,

EDUCATING YOUR DOCTOR

Unfortunately, it has been shown many times over in the past several decades that medical doctors are not trained in nutrition and many are unfamiliar with plant-based diets. When you go to your doctor, they may be skeptical and wary about your dietary changes. Some may even try to talk you out of choosing to eat a healthy diet. A plant-based-diet mom asked us at the T. Colin Campbell Center for Nutrition Studies for advice on how to better interact with her pediatrician, who was giving her a hard time for not feeding her children dairy foods. This was my response.

"Unfortunately, you are not alone in your frustrations with experiencing a doctor's lack of familiarity with a whole-food, plant-based diet. And while your doctor may need some education on plant-based nutrition, lecturing your doctor on nutritional science during a visit will not be productive for either of you. Pediatricians, particularly, are often active proponents of dairy foods and a standard 'varied' diet. As a family doc with pediatrics training, I can tell you that this is the dietary message we are taught to deliver. I would suggest the following brief, nonthreatening, non-science, pleasant response (assuming it applies to your family):

"'Our family has really been focusing on loading up with nutrient-rich fruits, vegetables, and whole grains. We aren't eating a lot of processed foods or refined foods, so we know that we are getting enough protein, calcium, fat, and iron from healthy plant sources like beans and leafy vegetables. This really seems to be working for us and we're going to stick with it for now. We [say however it was that you learned about the diet], and if you're interested we'd be happy to bring the information in to get your opinion on it because we value your opinion. If there's anything you think we should be checking (iron levels, blood count, B_{12}), we'd want to hear about this.'

"If this dietary friction continues to be a sore spot and you feel hassled and unsupported, I would search for a new doctor, especially if you have a lot of kids!"

of course, is to weigh yourself regularly. If you want to lose weight, you'll find that a whole-food, plant-based dietary pattern leads to weight loss without your having to limit your overall food intake. Eat as much of the approved foods as you want and you will lose weight. Weigh yourself regularly. This type of monitoring will help you stick with the plan. The other easy way to monitor your dietary pattern is with cholesterol tests. I suggest you get a blood cholesterol panel prior to your dietary shift. After as little as 2 weeks on your new diet—if you follow it strictly—you'll see improvements in your levels. If you check your cholesterol now, during the preparation phase, and in 1 month, after you've really gotten into the diet, your improved numbers should offer you confidence and motivation to continue.

With your heart and head in the right place, with supportive people surrounding you, with your house free of bad food temptations, and with your doctor involved and monitoring you, you are now truly prepared to give a whole-food, plant-based diet your best shot.

Chapter 14

The Campbell Plan: In with the New

E very once in a while, I get to see an "aha" moment happen right in front of me. It is wonderful. Perhaps it comes after I have just talked to a patient about their odds of having a major heart-disease "event" or a stroke. I can see the wheels turning. There is a transition in thinking right before my eyes. Perhaps the patient still has young kids. They would never get on a bus that had a 1-in-10 chance of barreling to a fatal, fiery crash, but perhaps they've just heard that they have a 10 percent chance of having a life-altering heart attack or dying within the next 10 years. They hear that medical guidelines suggest starting medications, which all have side effects, medications that will likely need to be taken for the rest of their life. I tell them the real problem is the food, and the wheels start turning. It doesn't happen that often, quite frankly, because getting information alone doesn't change us that often. That's why the factors discussed in the last chapter, the ones on the scorecard, are so crucial. They go far beyond the facts and figures.

But when the wheels really do turn right in front of me, I start getting questions like "What do I eat? Do you have a food list? Do you have a shopping list?" And one of the more common questions I get when patients realize that I follow my own recommendations is "What do you eat?"

This chapter is not only about answering these questions for you, but more importantly about giving you the skills to perpetuate this new lifestyle on your own. You know the expression: Give a man a fish and you feed him for a day; teach a man to fish and you feed him for a lifetime. This chapter is about teaching you how to fish, so to speak, for healthy plant foods in the grocery store.

STAPLE FOODS TO HAVE ON HAND

In the last chapter I gave you the bad news: the foods you need to throw out. Now I want to give you the good news: the incredible range of new foods you should seek out to thrive on. This list could go on for the next 30 pages, but I'll keep it as simple as I can. I mention some brand names in this list, but have absolutely no personal financial stake in doing so.

The New Staples

Pastas

100% whole wheat pasta of any variety

Brown rice pasta: Tinkyada is a brand I like that is commonly sold in the gluten-free section of grocery stores.

Whole Grains and Legumes

Oatmeal: The "old-fashioned" kind with nothing added

Regular brown rice: Any of the many different types, such as short, medium, or long grain or basmati; I enjoy Nishiki premium medium-grain brown rice.

Purple Thai rice or Chinese black rice: These have a nice look and a unique, nutty taste that's good for special occasions.

Instant brown rice: For when you don't have much time

Quinoa: Cooks fast

Whole wheat couscous: Cooks very fast

Beans! Most varieties are available dried, in bags, but need to be soaked overnight before cooking. Lentils of various types are available in bags and cook quickly. Because of my busy schedule, I often use canned beans, which I always have on hand.

Boxed Cereals

There is no more confusing aisle in the grocery store than the cereal aisle, full of packages with misleading labels. I'll admit that only the boring boxed cereals are healthy, but if you add some raisins and a banana and other fruits, you won't miss a thing. I recommend using oats as your breakfast base (see page 201 for my easy homemade muesli) because even the boring cereals have a lot of sodium. For convenience you might try these brands (or the generic versions):

Post Grape-Nuts   General Mills Chex

Post Bran Flakes   General Mills Kix

Post Shredded Wheat   General Mills Total

General Mills Cheerios

Or any other cereal with no added oil and less than 5 or 6 g sugar per serving

Breads/Crackers

100% whole grain bread: Food for Life's Ezekiel 4:9 is a particularly good sprouted grain bread found in the frozen health-food section of stores; there are many different products in the line.

Whole grain tortillas: Ezekiel 4:9 is good; La Tortilla Factory's Sonoma is also a good brand, as are Trader Joe's Corn & Wheat and plain corn tortillas. Take care to avoid tortillas with oil, which are very common.

Crackers: Wasa makes oil-free varieties of crackers. These are better with toppings and dips.

Rice thins: Some brands make small, circular thin rice crackers without oil.

Crackers and pretzels: Any variety of Mary's Gone Crackers gluten-free, oil-free, whole grain crackers or pretzels, available online in many flavors

Tortilla chips: La Reina brand unsalted, baked organic corn tortilla chips, available online

Baking

100% whole wheat pastry flour

Individual snack-size containers of 100% applesauce, unsweetened

Raisins

Dates

Basic spices: cinnamon, nutmeg

Baking soda and baking powder

Parchment paper: Not a food, obviously, but very useful for oil-free baking and roasting

Root Vegetables

Sweet potatoes and yams

White potatoes

Onions

Ginger: If you use this infrequently, peel a whole gingerroot, freeze it, and then grate it as needed.

Garlic: If you prefer fresh

Any other of the dozens of root vegetables that store well and have been used all over the world as reliable, stable sources of nutrition. This is a huge group of foods you can explore. How about trying taro? Fennel? Rutabaga? Cassava?

Jarred Sauces/Dressings

Tomato pasta sauces: Be careful; most premade pasta sauces have lots of oil and salt and frequently have added meat and cheese. Choose sauces that do not list oil in the ingredients. You can make your own or stock up on the couple of brand options that are more benign:

Ragú Light Tomato and Basil Pasta Sauce

Enrico's Traditional Pasta Sauce, oil free, no salt added

Trader Joe's Organic Spaghetti Sauce with Mushrooms

Salsas: Enrico's has no added salt or oil in a variety of styles. Look for low- or no-added-salt salsas.

Balsamic vinegar: We are very fortunate to have the F. Oliver's chain of stores where I live, which carries wonderful aged and flavored balsamic vinegars that are good for topping greens, salads, and many other foods. They offer their products online as well. Several other chains and businesses now offer the same types of vinegars.

Other vinegars: White, apple cider, rice vinegar, others as called for in recipes

Fat-free salad dressings: Be very careful with these. It's better to make your own dressings, as most fat-free dressings are basically flavored corn syrup with other added sugars, but some might be available with 3 or fewer grams of added sugar per serving. Look for a variety that does not list a sugar or syrup as the first ingredient and has less than 30 calories per 2-tablespoon serving.

Lemons and limes: Usually part of sauces and dressings. Good for seasoning greens and other recipes.

Canned Goods

Beans! Low-sodium varieties like great Northern beans, garbanzo beans (chickpeas), kidney beans, black beans, pinto beans, and *many* others

Diced tomatoes: Low- or no-sodium varieties

Tomato paste: If you don't want to throw out half a can of paste each time you use a little in a recipe, scoop it out into ice cube trays (which are about 1 tablespoon per cube), cover with plastic wrap, and freeze. After they're frozen, transfer the cubes to a freezer-safe container. They keep well for a long time.

Refrigerator Foods

Minced garlic: The chefs out there will prefer mincing their own fresh garlic, but for me and other lazy cooks, a big container of minced garlic is absolutely required.

Minced ginger: Same as garlic. Be careful to avoid ones with added salt and sugar.

Hummus: Like fat-free dressings, it can be difficult to find premade hummus that isn't loaded with tahini (ground sesame seeds) and oil. It's better—and far cheaper—to make your own (see the recipe on page 210), but if you can find it premade without oil or tahini, buy it and have it on hand for snacking. Oasis Mediterranean Cuisine makes a no-tahini, no-oil hummus.

Nondairy milk substitute: I prefer unsweetened almond milk. Beware of types that have lots of sugar. Stick with varieties with less than 5 grams of sugar per serving. Almond Breeze unsweetened almond beverage is available online.

Always have fresh, dark leafy greens on hand. Many are sold prewashed and prechopped.

Ground flaxseed: A great source of omega-3 ALA fat that can be used as a topping for oatmeal or even an egg replacer for baking

Tofu: Many recipes use blended silken tofu to create a creamy consistency. You can buy it in shelf-stable packages for longer storage. Extra-firm or firm tofu is good occasionally in stir-fry or scrambled tofu–type dishes.

Many other vegetables, depending on your meals for the week (you'll get a handle on this group when we discuss your shopping list for the next 2 weeks).

Frozen Foods

Chopped frozen greens

Frozen vegetable mixes: The many varieties available make it easy to make meals of many types, like Asian stir-fry, Southwestern (with beans), and others.

Frozen corn

Shelled, organic edamame: A fast snack in the microwave

Spices/Flavorings

Nutritional yeast: This is frequently used as a cheese replacement in recipes and in pasta.

Many others: It is important to have a wide selection of spices, which you will collect as you try more recipes. This is where you will find greater and greater enjoyment in your whole-food, plant-based diet. You'll cook with many more flavors than you might have previously. Buy by weight from bulk sections or natural-food stores so you can try new spices cheaply and get as little as you want.

You'll notice a few things missing from this list of staples. There are no prepared frozen meals or cheese or meat substitutes. These vegan convenience foods can be useful in your kitchen now and then, but many of them are highly refined and often have added salt, sugar, or fat. Despite the less than optimal nutrition, I sometimes suggest them as a means to transition away from the meat-, dairy-, oil-, and sugar-laden standard American diet. They can be regarded as steps in the right direction, like the restaurant

BEVERAGES

1. Water is the best thing to drink. It can improve your bowel habits, reduce headaches, and reduce kidney stones. I'm not sure there is conclusive evidence about the amount you should drink, but 8 glasses a day seems reasonable, if arbitrary.

2. Avoid fruit juices and sodas and artificially sweetened drinks. These are all loaded with sugar or, in the case of artificial sweeteners, will trigger your sugar addiction.

3. Alcohol is okay in small amounts, but for a great many of us it can be a big problem. Higher-risk drinking is more than 7 drinks a week for women and more than 14 drinks a week for men. "Higher risk" isn't just a reference to alcoholism; it means you are putting yourself at risk for a wide range of related diseases, like depression, insomnia, certain cancers, obesity, high blood pressure, gastrointestinal problems, and others. If you are even getting close to these cutoffs, I strongly suggest you consider cutting back. For optimal weight loss, avoid all alcohol.

food list in Chapter 4, but you will not experience significant health benefits until you move beyond the vegan/vegetarian high-fat, high-salt, high-sugar convenience foods.

As you expand the flavors and foods you enjoy, check out your local ethnic grocery stores. Some sell largely packaged food you should avoid, but many sell delicious, fresh, inexpensive produce varieties, some of which you may never have tried. For example, our local Asian market has interesting, affordable greens and nice rices, and our local Indian and Middle Eastern markets have bulk spices and healthy whole grains, like whole wheat pita and bulgur.

Substitutions

You have the staples now, but what do you do about eggs? Oils? Cheeses? How do you cook this new food and find substitutes for those things? This is a common question, particularly when people are first starting to change. It's typical to simply look for alternative ingredients for the same types of recipes and cooked foods you're used to. After all, that's familiar and easy, right? As you get more used to eating a whole-food, plant-based diet, you'll find that your tastes change. It will become less important to try to adapt your old habits to plant-based techniques because you simply won't be interested in the old habits anymore!

That being said, it can be very handy to know some basic techniques so you can use some of your current recipes and cookbooks to make healthier foods. With that in mind, see the table on pages 160 to 161 for the most important substitutions and techniques you need to know to start a healthier life.

TACKLING THE GROCERY STORE AND READING LABELS

In order to keep your kitchen safe and healthy and your habits good, you must do your best work at the grocery store. If you only bring good food home, you will have an easy time with this diet because there will not be any temptation to refuse or willpower required to avoid anything bad at home. Remember: Willpower is fragile and limited, but mindless habits are forever. Your choices at the grocery store are going to either make or break your mindless habits during the rest of the week. In this way, the time you spend in the grocery store is probably the single most important time of the week for your health.

Step 1: Eat before you go to the grocery store. Do not go to the grocery store hungry. In a study[1] of simulated shopping after fasting for 5 hours, people were likely to buy more calorie-dense foods. Further, people who shop from 4:00 to 7:00 p.m. tend to buy more high-calorie foods than do people who shop from 1:00 to 4:00 p.m.,[1] perhaps because those shopping earlier in the day are less hungry, having just had lunch. Maybe you've noticed this in yourself. When you go to the grocery store hungry, the prepared junk and the sugary and fatty stuff look much more tempting. Don't go to the store hungry. Eat at least a snack beforehand, and if possible, structure your day so you can go to the store after a meal.

Step 2: The most important section of the store is the produce section. Don't go to the "health" or "natural" section to become more healthy or natural; go to the produce section. Of course, you will go into the health-foods section for a few ingredients, but know that many of the items you'll see there are junky, processed foods with pretty pictures and confusing labels. After the produce section and the health section, you might spend time in the canned vegetables aisle, the pastas and sauces aisle, the cereal

(continued on page 166)

Trading In the Old for the New

INSTEAD OF THIS	USE THIS
Cow's milk	Any nondairy "milk," like soy milk or almond milk. For use on cereal or for drinking, use unsweetened almond milk. For baking, full-fat soy milk has a thicker texture, but you can use any nondairy milk.
Scrambled eggs	Scrambled tofu with LOTS of tasty spices and added veggies (see the recipe on page 200)
Eggs (for baking)	Any of these (each equal to 1 egg): 1. 1 tablespoon ground flaxseed mixed with 3 tablespoons water 2. Ener-G egg replacer (a starch powder you mix with water, as directed on the box) 3. $\frac{1}{2}$ mashed banana (optional: add $\frac{1}{2}$ teaspoon extra baking powder to avoid making the food denser) 4. $\frac{1}{4}$ cup plain tofu pureed in a food processor
Oils (for stove-top cooking)	Sorry! You are going to have to lose your taste for the heavy, coat-every-inch-of-your-mouth-and-arteries-with-an-oil-slick texture that is common to many standard foods and you usually have to chase with your favorite heartburn pill. You just won't be able to substitute anything healthy that gives the same texture. In fact, in time, you will come to consider that texture gross, like swishing with motor oil by accident. Trust me. For stove-top cooking and sautéing, use nonstick cookware and a few tablespoons of water or vegetable stock instead of an oil, and without sacrificing taste.
Pure fats, such as oils, butter, and margarine (for baking)	You have a couple of choices. Fruit purees are surprisingly good for baking, but they change the food's texture. They are particularly good for making soft baked goods like muffins, breads, and soft cookies. 1. Prune paste. Puree $\frac{1}{2}$ cup pitted prunes with $\frac{1}{4}$ cup water and use about $\frac{1}{3}$ of the amount of fat called for. For 1 stick butter ($\frac{1}{2}$ cup), use $\frac{1}{4}$ cup prune paste. Err on the side of undercooking, since baked goods become dry faster when you use fruits instead of fats. 2. Unsweetened applesauce. This is easy because it comes packaged in snack-size containers. Use a little less applesauce than the amount of fat that's called for: for $\frac{1}{2}$ cup fat, use $\frac{1}{3}$ cup applesauce. For $\frac{1}{3}$ cup oil, use $\frac{1}{4}$ cup applesauce. For amounts smaller than that, use a 1:1 swap. 3. Use nonstick and silicon baking materials. Parchment paper is great for oil-free cooking. Rarely, I use a little oil cooking spray and then wipe most of it off to avoid sticking. One small can lasts me several years.

INSTEAD OF THIS	USE THIS
Cheese	This is another tough one. I promise that you will lose your taste for pizza with $1/2$-inch-thick cheese and enough grease to soak through several napkins. (What do you think that's doing to your arteries, anyway? I'll tell you—it's destroying them!) There are vegan cheese replacements, but most are simply refined oils congealed with refined starches. I consider them unhealthy and unnatural and to be avoided.
	Vegan cookbooks commonly use cashew cheese sauce that gets fat from the nuts and "cheesy" flavor from nutritional yeast. This is tasty, but it's also a very-high-fat concoction that might sabotage your health goals. There are healthier varieties of creamy and cheesy sauces, but use nut sauces sparingly. Nutritional yeast flakes can be used to top pasta like a Parmesan cheese, but this is not a perfect cheese substitute.
Ground beef	As you've seen, I'm not crazy about meat substitutes, but I think that judicious use of plant-based alternatives is sometimes tasty in dishes calling for ground beef as a minor ingredient, like vegetable chili.
	Gimme Lean's replacement foods are tasty.
	TVP, or textured vegetable protein, is a more basic substitute that serves the purpose, as well.
Meat	You can buy substitutes if you're struggling with the transition, but if you find yourself eating lunches of vegan "cold cuts," vegan "cheese," and vegan "mayonnaise," you really haven't done anything good for your health.
Salad dressings	See pages 213 and 216. Also, try a flavored, aged balsamic vinegar, as mentioned in the Staples section. You may be able to find low-sugar, oil- free packaged dressings, but these are few and far between. If you find one and it tastes good, go for it.
Breakfast cereals	Oatmeal with fruit, raisins, ground flaxseed, and a few walnuts
Breads	100% whole grain breads
Ice creams	Frozen Banana Cream (page 246) is tasty and healthy and can be made with different fruits and many different toppings. You can make this using an affordable appliance called Yonanas.
	Fruit sorbet is extremely sugary, so it should be enjoyed judiciously.
	Soy ice creams should be minimally used, but they are available.

What Is This Food?

Read the ingredient list, usually found just below the Nutrition Facts table. The ingredients are listed in order of descending predominance by weight, starting with the most predominant component and going down to least predominant. To illustrate, let us say that an imaginary ingredient list says the product includes corn syrup, water, and strawberry flavoring. From this we know that, by weight, there is more corn syrup than water and more water than strawberry flavoring.

Once you have read the ingredient list, ask yourself two questions to determine which of the three food groups it belongs to:

Is this a whole food?

Is this a plant or animal?

If you can say that the food is mostly a whole food and a plant, then you are all set—it is a good food and can go into your cart. There is one caveat: Some whole plants are very calorie-dense because they are mostly fat, like nuts and seeds, avocados, coconuts, and olives. There are lots of wonderful nutrients in these foods, but people who are trying to cut their cravings for fat, reverse heart disease, or lose weight can sabotage their efforts by overconsuming these whole plants. Extremely high-fat plants should be used sparingly, depending on your circumstances and goals. For example, I've prescribed gorp (good old raisins and peanuts) as a snack when a patient is just beginning to contemplate a change from their daily drive-through junk meals. On the other hand, if you have advanced heart disease and have been told by the cardiologist to go home and prepare your will, you should avoid all high-fat plants, including peanuts. I want you to lose that craving for fat so thoroughly that oils and other high-fat foods never again tempt you.

Sometimes it can be hard to tell whether a food is whole or not. I find the most confusing category of foods to be grains. Which one of those grains is a whole food? The short answer is that the ingredient must say "whole," or else it is refined. The table on the opposite page has more details.[2]

WHOLE OR NOT? THE GRAINS

	WHOLE	REFINED
Wheat	Whole wheat, whole durum, bulgur, whole white wheat (a wheat variety called "white wheat")	Semolina, durum wheat, wheat, wheat flour, enriched flour
Rye	Whole rye, rye berries	Rye, rye flour
Oats	Essentially all oats and oat flours; often steamed, flattened, and/or rolled during processing to make them cook faster (quick-cook oats), but they contain the whole grain, whether old-fashioned, quick-cook, or steel-cut	
Rice	Brown rice, most other colored rices (black, red, purple), wild rice	White rice, rice
Corn	Whole corn flour, whole cornmeal, popcorn, masa, hominy (the last two being somewhat processed, but mostly whole)	Cornmeal, white and yellow corn flour, degerminated flour
Barley	Hulled barley, whole barley	Pearled barley
Amaranth	All	
Millet	All	
Quinoa	All	
Teff	All	
Spelt	Whole spelt	Spelt flour, spelt
Buckwheat (not wheat or even a grain, but commonly found with the grains in stores)	All	

Source: Whole Grains Council. Whole grains A to Z. n.d.
http://wholegrainscouncil.org/whole-grains-101/whole-grains-a-to-z.

Assess the Added Fat, Salt, and Sugar

At this point, the only thing we know about the food is what type of food it is. If the label says, "Whole wheat flour, olive oil, corn syrup, flavoring," then we know that by weight there is more whole wheat flour than olive oil and more oil than corn syrup, but we don't know if the manufacturer added lots of oil and sugar or just tiny bits. So now we have to peek at the numbers on the nutrition label.

Note: To follow a heart-disease-reversal diet, any food listing "oil" is off-limits.

Added fat. In general, a whole-food, plant-based diet with zero added fat will average out to have about 10 percent of its calories from fat, unless it consists of large amounts of high-fat plants. That means that when you look at a food label, any food containing more than 10 percent fat likely has a larger amount of either a high-fat plant or added oil. Look at the food's total calories per serving and do the math to figure out what 10 percent of that is (move the decimal one place to the left). Is the number of calories from fat higher than that? Lower? If it's higher than 10 percent and there is oil in the food, beware.

Added salt. Look at the sodium content. Ideally, the number of milligrams of sodium should be no higher than the number of calories. The upper limit of salt intake is suggested to be 2.3 grams per day.[3] Though there is uncertainty in the details, consuming more than this may contribute to high blood pressure (and therefore heart attack and stroke), poor bone health, and kidney stones.[3] All of these are related to complex activities taking place in the kidney and involve other minerals like potassium and calcium. So if you eat less than 2.3 grams per day of sodium and you eat about 2,000 to 2,300 calories a day, then some simple math shows you that you should have about the same number of milligrams of daily sodium intake as you do daily calories. If the food you are looking at has higher sodium than calories, you'd better also be eating lots of no-salt-added foods to bring down your average sodium intake.

Added sugar. This is a tough one because there is no hard and fast rule to follow. I hope the pending update to the Nutrition Facts label makes this easier to assess. I suggest you minimize added sugar. Sugar can sneak into your diet in a wide variety of ways identifiable by specific chemical names like fructose, dextrose, lactose, and glucose that in processed form go by names like syrups, nectars, and honey, as well as healthier-sounding names like fruit concentrates and cane juice. Be sure that added sugar is not a primary ingredient of the food. To assess exactly how much sugar is in a food demands a bit of math in your head, so you can skip it if you want. But if you want to try, multiply the number of grams of sugar by 4. That will give you the total number of calories provided by sugar. Then divide that number by the total number of calories per serving. Less than 5 percent of your total calories should be from added sugar. Whole fruits have much more than 5 percent sugar overall and are healthy, but don't have any *added* sugar. Avoid totally the obvious added-sugar foods like candies and processed desserts. Avoid sports drinks and fruit juices and sodas.

aisle, and the "ethnic" aisle, where you probably can find some delicious grains and beans. Then take a quick trip to the frozen section to stock up on frozen fruits and veggies. And that is it. That is my typical trip through the store, hitting the most useful parts. Stay out of the junk-food aisles altogether. Why look at sports drinks, sodas, cookies, and potato chips? You no longer eat or drink those, right?

Step 3: Become a Nutrition Facts connoisseur. As I write this, the FDA is in the process of revising food labels, so changes will be coming. Of course, for many of the healthiest foods, there are no labels. The fruits and veggies in the produce section don't have labels unless they are packaged in some way. Not having a label is a good sign that you're eating real food. For everything else, you're stuck with reading the labels. Regardless of what the FDA's next food label might look like, there are important principles that will help you separate good foods from bad foods, as shown on pages 162 to 165.

Now you know what should be in your kitchen, some of the basic substitutions and techniques, and how to read labels and shop at the grocery store. If you take these guidelines to heart—particularly those on using food labels to choose whole plant foods and minimize added salt, sugar, and fat—you will have all the nutritional knowledge you need to have the best health of your life. In the next chapter, we will put this all into action as we go over the details of the 2-week Campbell Plan trial.

Chapter 15

The Campbell Plan Menu Plan and Shopping List

Generally, people eat a small number of dishes regularly when they cook at home. Every once in a while, one of the dishes gets tiresome and you let it go and find another. Convenience and ease of preparation are crucial. Given the lack of variety in most of our lives, I am usually a bit overwhelmed by the menu plans included in many diet books. There are sometimes a bewildering variety of foods and dishes proposed for each day, way more than I would ever think of preparing. My wife, Erin Campbell, MD, MPH, and I are both extremely busy. Who wants to make two or three things to eat for every meal, three times a day?

With this in mind, I propose a meal plan that has realistic options for the busy reader but enough variety to give you many different cooking options over the next 2 weeks. This meal plan is a collection of recipes from Erin and me along with recipes from my favorite chefs and cookbooks. I strongly recommend that you buy a few cookbooks to help you improve your diet. The authors I have chosen to include in the Campbell Plan 2-week menu plan have easy-to-find cookbooks and Web sites that I recommend to all of my patients who are interested in being healthier. Use these next 2 weeks to sample my favorite recipe sources. All have been vetted by me, so you know their recipes are safe. Then go support these authors as you continue your transition.

These are my favorite recipe creators and contributing resources, presented in the order of how many recipes they contributed.

LeAnne Campbell, PhD

THE CHINA STUDY COOKBOOK (BENBELLA BOOKS)

Based on the principles in *The China Study,* LeAnne (my sister) created many delicious family-friendly recipes to feed her two healthy, hungry, athletic boys.

Lindsay S. Nixon

THE HAPPY HERBIVORE (BENBELLA BOOKS)

EVERYDAY HAPPY HERBIVORE (BENBELLA BOOKS)

HAPPY HERBIVORE LIGHT & LEAN (BENBELLA BOOKS)

I often highlight Lindsay's name as a go-to resource for all my patients because she has a true talent for creating familiar, tasty, easy recipes. She offers a meal plan service at www.getmealplans.com.

Cathy Fisher

STRAIGHTUPFOOD.COM

Cathy has been a culinary instructor for the leaders of healthy eating for many years. Her free Web site (www.StraightUpFood.com) is aptly named, with tons of recipes for delicious foods free of added salt, oils, and sugar.

Ann Esselstyn

CHEF DEL'S PREVENT AND REVERSE HEART DISEASE, BY CALDWELL B. ESSELSTYN JR., MD (AVERY)

If you have heart disease or any of its risk factors, *Prevent and Reverse Heart Disease* is the one book you must own. Get more information at www.dresselstyn.com.

Del Sroufe

CHEF DEL'S BETTER THAN VEGAN (BENBELLA BOOKS)

Chef Del is one of the great success stories of a whole-food, plant-based diet. After gaining lots of weight on a vegan junk-food diet, he lost more than 200 pounds by switching to a whole-food, plant-based diet. He has written an excellent cookbook that is optimal for weight loss as well as disease reversal.

Susan Voisin

FATFREE VEGAN KITCHEN

This is another wonderful free Web site (blog.fatfreevegan.com) with recipes for a wide variety of healthy foods. Stick to the recipes on Susan's blog, because some of the submissions on the related Web site have oil.

Keep in mind that you only need to find a handful of dishes that you enjoy to begin with. This will be the small cadre of meals you can cycle through in the beginning as you work on expanding your tastes.

I am certainly not a fancy chef. Though my wife likes to cook, we are both so busy that convenience is paramount. We often end up eating in the same basic pattern. For example, weekday breakfasts are usually cold cereal, oatmeal, or homemade muesli with fruit and unsweetened almond milk. Lunch is almost always leftovers, which are easy to reheat and eat at work. Snacks are fruits, breads, and hummus. Dinners are usually one-pot meals requiring minimal preparation and a very simple veggie side, usually steamed greens.

I know many people are similarly busy, so my wife and I have put several convenience options in our meal choices. We tried to schedule the more complicated recipes on the weekends, when you might have more time. Leftovers are absolutely fine, but instead of writing "Leftovers" for every lunch, we did include several lunch recipes. But eating leftovers is the easy, tasty thing to do, as noted above. Lunch recipes can be shifted to dinner if you need faster preparation.

You may note a greens theme; every single day should include dark, leafy greens. A few raw leaves on your sandwich do not count. You can eat vastly more greens if you steam them or cook them into another food. This should be a daily goal.

With its emphases on convenience, greens, and simplicity, here is a 2-week menu plan. Following the menu plan is a shopping list with everything you need for all of the dishes listed in the first 3 days. This will give you a great start on your journey.

MENU PLAN

DAY 1 | *Sunday*

BREAKFAST

Dr. Campbell's Muesli (p. 201)

LUNCH

Traditional Low-Fat Hummus sandwich (p. 210)

DINNER

Easy Spinach and Mushroom Lasagna (p. 222)

Optional: Salad of mixed greens, tomatoes, cucumbers, and shredded carrots topped with balsamic vinegar

Frozen Banana Cream (p. 246)

DAY 2 | *Monday*

BREAKFAST

Quick Stove-Top Oatmeal (p. 198)

LUNCH

Leftover Easy Spinach and Mushroom Lasagna
or
Tasty Tostados (p. 208)

Whole fruit of your choice

DINNER

Quick Three-Bean Soup (p. 224)

Fiesta Corn Bread (p. 228)

Steamed Kale (p. 229)

DAY 3 | *Tuesday*

BREAKFAST

Dr. Campbell's Muesli (p. 201)

LUNCH

Leftover Quick Three-Bean Soup
or
Traditional Low-Fat Hummus sandwich (p. 210)

Whole fruit of your choice

DINNER

Pineapple Stir-Fry (p. 234) over brown rice

Sautéed Bok Choy (p. 230)

Banana-Maple Oatmeal Cookies (p. 246)

DAY 4 | *Wednesday*

BREAKFAST

Slow-Cooker Oatmeal (p. 199)

LUNCH

Quick Burgers (p. 209)

DINNER

Burrito Bar (p. 235)

Steamed Kale (p. 229) with Miraculous Walnut Sauce (p. 240)

Fruit salad

DAY 5 | *Thursday*

BREAKFAST

Tofu Scramble (p. 200) made with leftover Burrito Bar veggies

100 percent whole grain toast

LUNCH

Easy Pasta Salad (p. 211)
or
Leftover Burrito Bar

Whole fruit of your choice

DINNER

Dr. Campbell's Bachelor Meal (p. 236)

Chocolate No-Bake Cookies (p. 247)

DAY 6 | *Friday*

BREAKFAST

Dr. Campbell's Muesli (p. 201)
or
100 percent whole grain, low-sugar boxed cereal with berries

LUNCH

Leftover Dr. Campbell's Bachelor Meal
or
Zucchini Pritti-Hummus Wrap (p. 210)

Whole fruit of your choice

DINNER

Rice with Salsa, Beans, and Cilantro (p. 223)

Sautéed Baby Spinach (p. 232)

Fruit salad

DAY 7 | *Saturday*

BREAKFAST

The BEST Banana Bread (p. 202) with low-sugar,
100 percent fruit jam

Cardamom-Raisin Rice Pudding (p. 203)

LUNCH

Ocean Chickpea Sandwiches (p. 214)

Sweet Potato Fries (p. 219)

DINNER

Minestrone Soup (p. 225) with 100 percent whole grain bread

Global Greens (p. 230)

Pineapple Sponge Cake (p. 245)

DAY 8 | *Sunday*

BREAKFAST

Panana Cakes (p. 204)

Berry Sauce (p. 205)

LUNCH

Leftover Minestrone Soup
or
Hearty Everything Salad (p. 215)

Vinaigrette of your choice (p. 213 or 216) or balsamic vinegar

Whole fruit of your choice

DINNER

Fabulous Sweet Potato Enchiladas (p. 237)

Rainbow Greens (p. 233)

DAY 9 | *Monday*

BREAKFAST
Dr. Campbell's Muesli (p. 201)

LUNCH
Leftover Fabulous Sweet Potato Enchiladas
or
Ensalada Azteca (p. 216)

Whole fruit of your choice

DINNER
Creamy Pasta and Broccoli (p. 238)

Sautéed Baby Spinach (p. 232)

DAY 10 | *Tuesday*

BREAKFAST
Quick Stove-Top Oatmeal (p. 198)

LUNCH
Leftover Creamy Pasta and Broccoli
or
Baked Tofu sandwiches: Baked Tofu (p. 218) with Vegan Mayo
(p. 214) on whole grain bread with tomatoes and baby spinach

Whole fruit of your choice

DINNER
Chili sans Carne (p. 226) over brown rice (rice is optional)

Steamed Kale (p. 229)

Mixed Fruit Cobbler (p. 248)

DAY 11 | *Wednesday*

BREAKFAST

Slow-Cooker Oatmeal (p. 199)

LUNCH

Baked Potatoes (p. 220) topped with leftover
Chili sans Carne

Whole fruit of your choice

DINNER

Garden Pizza (p. 240)

Sautéed Baby Spinach (p. 232)

DAY 12 | *Thursday*

BREAKFAST

Citrus-Infused French Toast (p. 207)

Berry Sauce (p. 205)

LUNCH

Simple Chopped Salad (p. 212) with whole wheat pitas

Whole fruit of your choice

DINNER

Cumin-Infused Vegetables and Chickpeas
over Quinoa (p. 242)

Steamed Kale (p. 229)

DAY 13 | *Friday*

BREAKFAST

Dr. Campbell's Muesli (p. 201)

or

100 percent whole grain, low-sugar boxed cereal with berries

LUNCH

Leftover Cumin-Infused Vegetables and Chickpeas over Quinoa

or

Soba Peanut Noodles (p. 221)

Whole fruit of your choice

DINNER

Sloppy Lentil Joes (p. 243) on whole grain bread or brown rice

Salad of mixed greens, tomatoes, cucumbers, and
shredded carrots

DAY 14 | *Saturday*

BREAKFAST

Potato Scramble (p. 206)

100 percent whole grain toast

LUNCH

Mango-Lime Bean Salad (p. 217)

Traditional Low-Fat Hummus (p. 210)

Toasted 100 percent whole wheat pitas

DINNER

Pumpkin Gnocchi with Italian Vegetable Sauce (p. 244)

Sautéed Baby Spinach (p. 232)

Amazingly Delicious Date Fruit Pie (p. 250)

THE CAMPBELL PLAN
GROCERY SHOPPING LIST

This list is a little overwhelming, but we wanted to include every single item you will need to cook all the recipes for the first 3 days. Many of these items are staples that are used in a number of this book's recipes. They will last a long time before you need to buy them again.

FIRST 3 DAYS

Produce

Apples and/or citrus fruit

Avocado

Baby spinach

Bananas

Bell pepper, red

Berries

Bok choy, 1½ pounds

Cabbage, small

Carrots

Cilantro (optional)

Cucumber

Dark green lettuce

Garlic

Gingerroot

Green onions

Greens, mixed (optional)

Kale, large bag pre-washed, chopped or 2 small bunches

Lemons

Mushrooms, 8 ounces

Onions, yellow

Tomatoes

Grains, Spices and Herbs, and Baking Supplies

Almonds, sliced

Baking powder

Baking soda

Basil, dried

Brown rice

Cayenne pepper

Chia seeds (optional)

Cinnamon, ground

Cocoa powder

Cornmeal, yellow whole grain

Cornstarch

Cumin, ground

Dates, chopped

Egg replacer (optional)

Flaxseed, ground

Garlic powder

Lemon juice

Maple syrup

Nutritional yeast

Old-fashioned (rolled) oats, two 42-ounce packages

Onion powder

Oregano, dried

Paprika, smoked if available

Parsley, dried

Pepper, black, ground

Pepper, red, flakes

Raisins

Rosemary, dried

Salt (interchangeable with sea salt)

Sea salt (optional)

Sesame seeds (optional)

Steel-cut oats

Sucanat

Tarragon, dried

Vanilla extract

Walnuts

Whole wheat pastry flour

Packaged, Canned, and Frozen Foods

Applesauce, unsweetened

Asian hot sauce (optional)

Balsamic vinegar

Beans, black, low-sodium, canned

Beans, pinto, low-sodium, canned or fat-free refried beans

Beans, red kidney, low-sodium, canned

Black olives, sliced (optional)

Bread, 100 percent whole grain with no added oil

Brown rice vinegar or rice vinegar

Corn, frozen

Dijon mustard

Garbanzo beans, (chickpeas), low-sodium, two 15-ounce cans

Lasagna noodles, 100 percent whole wheat or brown rice

Nondairy milk, unsweetened, with no added oil (for the first 3 days, any nondairy milk can be used)

Orange juice

Pineapple, chunks, two 14- to 20-ounce cans

Roasted red peppers

Salad dressing, fat-free, low-sodium

Salsa, low-sodium

Soy sauce or tamari, low-sodium

Spaghetti sauce, oil-free, two 24-ounce jars

Spinach, 10-ounce frozen

Sweet red chili sauce

Tofu, reduced-fat firm or extra firm (not silken), two 15- or 16-ounce packages

Tomatoes, canned, no salt added, crushed with jalapeño chile peppers

Tortillas, whole grain, oil-free, gordita-style if available

Vegetable broth, low-sodium with no added oil

Vegetables, mixed, frozen

Chapter 16

The Campbell Plan for Life: Making It Stick

One of the recurring themes in dietary research is that even with initial success at behavior change, maintaining that behavior change is difficult. This is particularly true with diets. Think for a moment about the people surrounding you in your everyday life. Think of those who are not obese, meaning that they are of a healthy weight or just overweight (having a BMI of under 30). Which of these people do you think will gain weight in the future? There are many factors to consider, but one of the better predictors of weight gain is if someone is currently or recently has been on a diet with calorie restriction. Seventy-five percent of the studies in a review found that current or recent dieting predicts future weight gain among people who are not yet obese.[1]

Do not go on a calorie-restriction diet. You would be joining an unfortunate group of people who are likely to gain more weight in the long run.

As I mentioned in Chapter 13, I suggest you adopt a whole-food, plant-based lifestyle, make better food choices, and then simply don't worry about counting calories or reducing your food intake. In fact, if you are eating the way I suggest, you will be eating a significantly larger volume of food throughout the day. But just because you can eat all you want doesn't mean that you won't fall off the wagon and start sliding back into your old diet. You'll encounter different challenges, with different triggers, in each stage of your journey. Even though I'm asking you to engage in a short-term experiment with The Campbell Plan, let us talk through some of the opportunities you'll have to make this a lifelong lifestyle, so you can reap truly innumerable benefits.

THE SHORT TERM
(WEEKS TO A FEW MONTHS)

In the short run, you will find the main challenges result from changing your tastes and habits. Studies show that our preferences for fat and salt do change depending on what we eat. People who consume diets with less added fat actually have a reduced taste preference for fat.[2] It's like switching from whole or 2% milk to fat-free milk. At first the fat-free tastes watery and it takes some time to get used to it. After a while, though, the fat-free seems normal, and if you go back to whole milk it seems like it's excessively thick and creamy.

The same principles have been found to be true with salt consumption. People put on a low-sodium diet found that eventually they had a decreased preference for highly salted foods.[3]

How long did this take? In both studies, the people's taste preferences changed in about 12 weeks.[2,3] That certainly doesn't mean it doesn't start to happen sooner. It is likely that more significant changes in your diet will lead to faster taste adaptation. Interestingly, it was found that how often the food in question was consumed determined how much tastes changed, not the overall amount.[2] This leads to a useful tip: If you continue to eat refined plants and animal foods as frequently as you did before, but in smaller portions, you may not be helping yourself change your tastes. If you want to truly change your taste preferences, also decrease how frequently you consume those foods rather than focusing just on the amount.

During these first 3 months, you are not only waiting for your tastes for fat and salt to fully change, but also coping with the withdrawal caused by eating less sugar. We know that sugar has significant addictive properties. In fact, when rats are given lots of sugar and then it is taken away, they get anxious, aggressive, and have measurable changes in their physiology.[4]

This is why behavior change is hard work! The goal is to make new habits as quickly and healthfully as possible. Habits are ingrained and don't require a lot of mental or emotional energy. This is what makes them easy to maintain. The process of breaking these habits, though, requires some real work. You will need willpower.

What is willpower, anyway, and how can I help you along? In their excellent book *Willpower: Rediscovering the Greatest Human Strength,*[5] Roy Baumeister and John Tierney describe the many psychological experiments that led to a breakthrough in our understanding of will-power. In one study,[6] female participants were asked to watch the saddest part of a movie, when a dying woman says good-bye to the people she loves. Some of the women were told to watch this tearjerker while remaining as *neutral* as possible, both inside and out—no crying on the outside and no sadness on the inside. The other women in the trial were told to be as *natural* as possible. If they felt moved to, they could cry or feel sad.

Then all the participants undertook a separate task of tasting and rating ice cream. Unbeknownst to the women, the researchers didn't care at all about their taste ratings for the ice cream, but instead were measuring how much ice cream each participant ate. It turned out that the women

BOLSTERING WILLPOWER DURING THE EARLY TRANSITION

1. Have healthy foods available at all times. If you have a stressful day at work or home (and who doesn't?), know that this will drain your blood sugar and thus your willpower. All sorts of bad temptations will be more difficult to resist. Thwart the potential problem by eating healthy blood sugar boosters along the way. The best foods for a quick but healthy boost? Whole fruits.

2. Choose foods that will give you an even blood sugar level over a longer period of time. This is another reason to eat a whole-food, plant-based diet. Foods with lots of fiber (found only in plants) accomplish this naturally.

3. Eat a healthy snack or full meal before you go to the grocery store.

4. Do not let clouds of unfinished tasks hang over your head; it will drain your willpower.

5. Keep a clean living space to prevent clutter from draining your willpower. Research has shown that a clean room leads to healthier food choices.[7]

6. Keep your home environment as free of temptation as possible. Realize that every time you walk by a bag of greasy potato chips, even if you

who had just consciously restricted their emotions ate a lot more ice cream. In fact, they ate more than 50 percent more (211 grams versus 135 grams). This ice cream test is commonly used to assess self-control. So another way to describe this experiment is to say that the women who restricted their emotions had less self-control. Why? After all, the women who let their emotions flow during the movie actually began the ice cream task feeling sadder, if anything. They were in a more emotional state.

As it turns out, willpower is a resource that can be used up, like cash in your wallet. Furthermore, a variety of tasks can use it up, with all of them drawing from the same pool. As Tierney and Baumeister describe, intense thinking activities like making decisions can use up willpower, as can stifling emotions and resisting temptation.[5] Working all day at a demanding job in which you make stressful decisions leaves you with less willpower

resist opening it, you are still draining away your pool of willpower. Eventually you may cave, whether it's with the potato chips or a totally different temptation you would rather not indulge.

7. Recognize that you won't always be able to prevent yourself from giving in to temptations, but make yourself this promise: Every time you want an unhealthy food, you will eat something healthy first (a piece of whole fruit, for example), wait 15 minutes, and then indulge as you please. Chances are that more often than not, you will not get around to eating the bad food.

8. If you know you'll be walking into a situation where there will be triggers that might cause you to make an unhealthy choice, decide ahead of time how you are going to deal with it. For example, if you know that someone is bringing cookies to the office, plan to eat your fruit before you eat any cookies. Or if you're hungry and know you'll see a fast-food restaurant along your route, decide not to stop there and instead go to a nearby grocery store to get a healthier snack. Making a decision ahead of time and then sticking with it preserves willpower.

9. Keep your work environment as free of temptation as possible. Get that candy jar out of your office!

at the end of the day to resist temptations. So the women who were stifling their emotions were using up their pools of willpower.

How do you plug the drain your willpower seeps through throughout the day? Are we bound to be chasing temptations at the end of every difficult day? The surprising answer is that blood sugar plays an important role in helping you to maintain willpower. Stifling emotions, making difficult decisions, and stressing your brain all demand blood sugar. In studies, people who ate or drank something to raise their blood sugar levels could blunt the depletion of willpower or restore its supply.[5]

This leads to some useful strategies for use in the early stages of behavior change. You are still in that difficult position of having to resist temptations and don't yet have in place the great habits that will take care of you in the future, so use these strategies to improve your chances of success.

Take your health one day at a time. There is no need to be perfect or anxious. This should be a time of exploration and enjoyment. You will likely start to notice your tastes changing within weeks of changing your diet, and they will continue to change. The habits you form will become more and more stable and mindless, and the health benefits of your efforts will quickly start to emerge.

Let's not lose the forest for the trees, though. While we have been talking about overcoming difficulties that might arise, let me assure you that there's a good possibility that this will be the easiest, most wonderful health choice you have ever made. It makes me think of some of the patients who've been helped by it: A 30-year-old who had been reliant on heavy-duty heartburn medication since he was 14 no longer needed it after he changed his diet. It happened within weeks. The middle-aged marathoner who developed recurrent chest pain just jogging a very short distance met Dr. Esselstyn and adopted a heart-disease-reversal diet. Within weeks he noted decreased chest pain and avoided the open heart surgery he was scheduled for. The kid with asthma and chronic congestion whose mom came back to the clinic a month later to tell me her child no longer needed inhalers or decongestants and allergy medications.

In light of benefits like this, when you consider that you might require lifelong medication or be hospitalized for a dangerous procedure, the challenges of eating oatmeal for breakfast suddenly seem rather trivial, don't you think?

THE MEDIUM TERM
(THE FIRST MANY MONTHS)

As you conquer the early personal transition, you might find that there is one area that presents stubborn challenges—social environments that you have no control over.

Let's tackle a tough one: going to someone else's house to eat. This brings up a problem that manifests itself in a few different scenarios, as we'll see. The problem is this: Someone you like is putting a lot of effort into doing something nice for you by cooking a meal and hosting you, and demanding that they do it your way just seems extremely rude. Doing something like that certainly is not the way I was raised, and probably not the way you were, either. This situation is a tough one. There is no sugar-coating it.

This is a good time to take stock of who in your life is supportive. Who is inviting you over? Do they sincerely want to support your interests and your attempts to be healthier? If you are close friends or family and you know that these people sincerely care about you, go ahead and let them know that you are working with your doctor (which is what you should be doing, even if you are healthy and only getting screening tests) and changing your diet to improve your health. Let them know that it seems to be working, but there are certain rules you have to follow. Do not preach and do not belittle, even subtly, their lifestyle choices because they are different from the choices you have made. That *is* rude and obnoxious! Then suggest that you bring your own dish to share with everyone and follow through with a great dish and a nice present for the hosts.

Is this perfect? No. It doesn't automatically make it easy or erase the social challenges, but it is a respectful and responsible way to safeguard your health while protecting your relationships. In fact this may be less painful than you imagine. In one study, cooks who prepared vegetables with their meals were seen as more thoughtful and attentive and less lazy, boring, and self-absorbed.[8] In addition, having vegetables included in a meal actually increased the perception that the main dish would taste good.[8] You could provide a healthy, tasty vegetable main dish and be regarded as both the hero and a wonderful cook who improved all the other dishes.

But what if the dinner party or gathering is hosted by people you don't know well, or by people who do not support you? That is a shame, but it happens sometimes, like at a work-related event where you don't want to talk about your health choices at all. I encourage you to fundamentally explore why you are spending time with people who are oblivious or even hostile to your best interests and good health, but you can make new friends and acquaintances later. This time, you have to go. Here is what I want you to do: Just before going to the gathering, eat a healthy meal at home. Then go to the gathering and eat a second small "tasting" meal out of politeness if you have to. Load up on the side dishes, the salad, the veggies, and then, if you must, eat a small amount of the main dish.

As you've seen throughout the book, following this dietary pattern is not about being 100 percent anything. For those people *in good health* who are eating a whole-food, plant-based diet 90 to 95 percent of the time, I do not believe there to be an irrefutable weight of evidence to prove you will die or get terrible diseases from infrequently eating some animal foods or refined-plant foods. Go ahead and have some of the fish or seafood, and enjoy a taste of the dessert. For most hosts, seeing you eat a decently sized "taste" is enough to demonstrate appreciation for the work they have done for you.

Going out to dinner with friends is easier than the situations I've just described, because it is much easier (expected, actually) to ask restaurants to cater to your needs. There are very few restaurants that cannot provide enough food choices for a healthier plant-based meal. It's likely that you'll find a whole new set of restaurants you prefer over the old standard restaurants. This may put you slightly at odds with friends, but there usually is enough overlap in restaurant preferences for everyone to find something on a menu that they can enjoy.

Hosting is perhaps the easiest of all. As you learn more about the different whole-food, plant-based meals that are possible to make, you'll find plenty of recipes that appeal to just about everyone. There are sandwich types of finger foods, dips, breads, snacks, and main dishes that range from basic family favorites like lasagna to fancy dishes that fill the menus at high-end vegan restaurants, and cookbooks are available for every occasion. I do suggest making several dishes for people to eat rather than just one dish. That way, if they can't stand eating anything with tofu, for example, they have another option. More often than not, though, I see people try healthier versions of typical foods and not have any idea that they just ate something that was good for them. Unfortunately, people think healthy eating is tasteless eating, and this is your chance to show them how enjoyable it can be.

Discussing Your Choice

Doug Lisle, PhD, is a brilliant, well-known speaker and psychologist who has risen to national prominence by artfully explaining how to understand social interactions and health decisions in ways that anybody can understand. I strongly recommend reading a book he coauthored called *The Pleasure Trap: Mastering the Hidden Force That Undermines Health and Happiness*. He recommends what he calls the "seems" strategy when it comes to discussing your health choices with those around you.

What we choose to eat is intensely personal—sometimes oddly so, in my opinion. People feel very strongly about their food choices and know that those choices are important. When they hear that you are trying something totally different from their current standard diet, they may regard it at a very basic level as a threat to their status. Do you think you know something they don't? Are you suggesting their choices are bad? Are you taking actions to improve your health that they have been longing to do, but have been unable to?

In this way, in the hierarchy of our social circles, making a dramatically different food choice can be seen as a threat to someone's status. It may all be relatively unconscious, but it will be interpreted as a threat nonetheless. How does this manifest? In these typical comments and questions:

"Where do you get your protein [or iron or calcium, etc.]?"

"What in the world CAN you eat?" as if clearly the answer is "nothing."

"I thought about doing that but didn't because I need to be more athletic [or strong or muscular, etc.]."

"Eww. I could *never* live without meat [or dairy, etc.]."

"Plants feel pain, too, you know."

And as they eat their food, you may hear things like "Uh-oh, can I eat this in front of you?"

"Don't you want some of this?" as they point to their meat.

I feel that many times these types of comments are related to a rather primal feeling of a threat to status. Are you trying to move a notch above them in the social hierarchy?

So, as Dr. Lisle says, your response has to appropriately recognize what is happening and do everything you can to soothe them about this perceived threat. The "seems" strategy is a way to do this gently. Do not preach or suggest you know what is best (even if you do). Explain that this "seems" to be something you just wanted to try. You can say it "seems" to be working. You "seem" to be losing weight and "seem" to be feeling good. Heck! You can pretend you barely know what's going on, but who knows, maybe you'll do this diet a while longer! You certainly should not be apologizing for your new habits, but you should be reassuring them that this is not a threat. It is a soft issue. You are not going to point out their flaws or rub your improved health in their face. You are not going to try to change the person.

One of the interesting trends since *The China Study* was published is the change in the public perception of plant-based diets over the last 10 years, which has made these types of difficult conversations less common. Plant-based diets are becoming much more acceptable and recognized as a healthy lifestyle choice. At some point soon, we may reach a point where handling others' objections to your diet will be unnecessary. Like smoking became uniformly understood to be unhealthy, the standard American diet, including excessive amounts of animal foods and processed foods, will eventually be widely understood to be unhealthy.

For those of you in the early to middle stages of adopting a healthier diet, these social issues will be new. Your success will be much easier with social support, as was discussed in reference to the scorecard in Chapter 13. Ultimately, you want people in your life who care about you, respect you, and support you. You can deal with the difficult social situations for a long time, but after a while you might think about changing your scene, if you know what I mean. Particularly for those of you following the diet strictly because you have heart disease, a cancer diagnosis, or something equally serious, you must politely but firmly make your health the top priority. If people cannot accept your choice and allow you the space to live with it, it is time to find new people. This may be of benefit in more than one way. Recent research has shown that bad health outcomes, like being obese and having mental health problems, spread through social networks in a manner similar to the way a virus might.[9, 10] Basically, you are more likely to be unhealthy if your friends are unhealthy.

THE LONG TERM (MONTHS TO MANY YEARS)

Your tastes have changed, you have a bunch of great dishes that you love to eat, and you have habits in place so you never again have to rely just on willpower. Your family and social connections are supportive and stable. You feel comfortable with your choices and perhaps have been experiencing major health benefits for quite a long time. There is no turning back.

There are just a few tips to consider at this point, and again they involve challenges in eating away from home.

The first is eating out. It is easy to find tasty vegetarian meals at most places, but unfortunately, it can be difficult to find meals that are prepared without ample oil. Avoiding large amounts of oil is the single biggest challenge to eating out. For those who want to follow a heart-disease-prevention and -reversal diet, you will probably have to limit your culinary excursions to a few options. Generally, you can find steamed veggies at Asian restaurants and sometimes at Mexican restaurants as well. You can go to any restaurant that has a salad buffet, of course. To really avoid oil, you have to communicate to the waitstaff that you have a medical issue that means you cannot have oil; sometimes it works to say you have a serious allergy problem. Otherwise, I find, servers routinely ignore any request you make for not using oil, even when they nod as if to say they'll take care of it. In some circumstances, they may not know that premade sauces consist largely of oils.

For those who choose to minimize their intake of animal foods and processed plants rather than strictly avoiding them, the options are more wide ranging. The table in Chapter 4 that suggests what to order at restaurants can guide you in selecting foods anyplace in the country. While these are far from perfectly health-promoting foods, they often are tasty and convenient and better than most of the other options you can find.

In the past 10 years, the number of plant-based and plant-friendly restaurants has exploded, particularly in certain areas of the country. In most metropolitan areas there are numerous restaurants that are exclusively vegetarian or even vegan. Most other restaurants are now offering plant-based options that are interesting and appealing, far beyond the boring pasta primavera of old. You can even skip the meat and dairy at many fast-food restaurants now.

This makes traveling in the United States pretty tasty, easy, and exciting now. I love eating my way through a new city. There are usually more than enough options and places to try.

Another issue that comes up for families is when the kids eat away from home a lot. Kids, of course, eat away from home most days of the year, at school. The easiest thing to give them is leftovers that can be eaten at room temperature. Many of the foods in this book are actually tastier as leftovers, and are fine at room temperature. In addition you can always do the good old standby sandwiches, like peanut butter and jelly on whole wheat bread with natural peanut butter and low-sugar jelly (not artificially sweetened), or something like a tofu sandwich with fresh veggies and mustard, or a hummus sandwich or tomato sandwich with salt and pepper and cucumbers. Pack some whole fruits and some homemade cookies, maybe a side of bean or pasta salad to really fill them up. There are lots of choices, and you'll find some that your kids love.

Some people worry about their kids not fitting in with the other kids. Kids can be ruthless, and no one wants their kid to be picked on. But remember that with kids, most "cool" things start out as something a little bit different or new, but then there's a champion of it who makes it cool. If your kids are comfortable, confident, and don't regard their food as a source of embarrassment, but rather something that will make them healthier and stronger, they'll convey that attitude to the other kids. The other kids may even want to trade lunches so they can try the more interesting foods. But actually, a plant-based diet does not need to be that strange. I eat lots of normal-looking food! I have seen several children go through this process in my own extended family. They were kids who were successful in school socially, intellectually, and athletically, at both small rural Southern schools and larger city schools. The food really isn't that big a deal socially unless you make it one, or unless there are preexisting issues (a bully is already targeting your kid, for example). Remember, you are setting your child up for lifelong healthy habits and tastes that will serve them well in innumerable ways for decades to come.

As you are settling in to a new lifestyle for the long term, I think it is worth pointing[11] out that the factors that predicted your success with your initial changes remain as important as ever. Every once in a while, go back to the scorecard, presented again below. Can you check off each factor, or do you need to focus on patching up some holes that have developed? If so, that's the most important thing you can do for continued success.

FACTORS PREDICTING SUCCESS IN CHANGING BEHAVIOR

1. You have clear, *personal* reasons that justify a *strong desire* to change the foods you eat.

2. You have *minimized obstacles* (environmental, cognitive, physical) to adopting a new dietary pattern.

3. You have the necessary *skills* and *confidence* to implement this new lifestyle.

4. You feel *positive* about your new dietary goals and believe they will be *beneficial*.

5. Your dietary goals are consistent with your *self-image* and *social norms*.

6. You have *support* and *encouragement* from people you value and a *community* that supports your dietary changes.

Certain things have been shown to help people stay on track. One is monitoring yourself. Whether you go in for a blood cholesterol test now and then, weigh yourself regularly, or keep a food diary for a week or two if you feel yourself starting to slip, these steps may help you be more conscious of and motivated to maintain your healthy lifestyle. Keep learning and finding ways to engage your heart and emotions in your social and family networks, your goals, and your motivation to continue this lifestyle.

THE FULL LIFESTYLE

I do consider this a lifestyle rather than just a diet. As you improve your diet, you will find that other parts of your life affecting your health become more important to you as well. This is a book about nutrition and food choices, but also vitally important for your health are exercise, sleep, and stress management, among other factors. All of these are connected.

Exercise can have wide-ranging benefits, helping your heart, your brain, your bones, your metabolism, your mood, and many other aspects of your health. Adults should get 150 minutes per week of moderate-intensity (brisk walking, for example) or 75 minutes per week of vigorous (jogging, for example) exercise. You can do this in small chunks of at least 10 minutes throughout the week. In addition, weight training, or resistance training involving all the major muscle groups in your body, should be done twice a week.

Having run several marathons, I am passionate about exercise. But as enthusiastic as I am about physical activity, I do not think any amount of exercise can overcome a bad diet, particularly for certain outcomes like heart disease. When I talk to people who are trying to lose weight, more often than not they are focusing on getting to the gym more often as their primary strategy. If they have even considered their diet, they are making what I consider to be minor changes, like eating more chicken. This strategy usually doesn't work for very long, if at all. On the other hand, I have had people lose weight on a whole-food, plant-based diet without any exercise at all. They accrue many other health benefits at the same time.

The bottom line is that exercise is extremely important and I encourage it heartily, but at the foundation of your healthy lifestyle needs to be the food you eat.

Sleep and stress also have been shown to be more important than people realize for short-term and long-term health outcomes. I see many people with poor sleep habits, often intertwined with mild depression or anxiety. As a starting point, I recommend adhering to good sleep hygiene behaviors to help with this. These include having relatively fixed waking and sleeping times every day, keeping your bedroom conducive to relaxation and sleep, avoiding naps, exercising regularly (preferably early in the day), avoiding alcohol and late-day meals, and other suggestions. Full recommendations can easily be found online with a simple search for "sleep hygiene." These practices are important and can play a role in our mental health as well.

And stress? Who can avoid that? How we deal with it can be important for our well-being. Dr. Ornish's program for reversing heart disease includes rather extensive meditation and yoga practice. If stress is thwarting your efforts to improve your health, it is definitely worth considering some of these stress-relieving practices.

All of these various lifestyle factors, and others, are integral to your health and happiness. However, I do believe that nutrition should be the foundation to your approach. If you are only going to work on one thing, it should be your diet. Because willpower is a resource that can be used up, I worry about people being too distracted by other lifestyle-related resolutions they've made when I see them struggling to adhere to a healthy diet. On the other hand, sometimes the more good you do for yourself in one area, the more good you feel like doing in other areas. Remember the rats I took to my grade school classroom? Those eating the diet that promoted lower cancer rates voluntarily exercised more throughout the day. In this way, these different lifestyle factors are not isolated, but rather integrated. Actions you take in one area may help you in another.

Chapter 17

Conclusion

There is a chasm between powerful nutrition and lifestyle information and the medical system's standards of care. Evidence-based nutrition is simply absent from the vast majority of our medical system. Intellectually, I knew this when I started my medical training. But emotionally I couldn't appreciate the consequences of this broken part of our medical system until I saw it right in front of me. It was a day early in my training when I met a patient who taught me this lesson (details insignificant to the meaning of the story have been altered to protect the patient's privacy).

On this particular day the resident physician overseeing me asked me to go see a woman with diabetes. The young doctor pulled me aside and told me this woman was in the later stages of her disease. She was losing a lot of protein in her urine and within the past year she had had bilateral "BKAs"—below-the-knee amputations. "She is near the end," the resident told me.

I knocked on the door and walked into the room to meet an overweight, middle-aged woman sitting in a large electric wheelchair that was taking up most of the limited space in the sterile exam room. I sat down and started asking her history: "When was your surgery?" "Have you been having any problems recently?" "What are you hoping to address at today's visit?" All the routine questions.

My lasting memory of that early interaction was a sense that this woman had been irreparably altered in the most profound of ways. She would never walk again. She could never again engage with the world with the ease that I did. Going grocery shopping, going outside, getting a job, cooking, going to the bathroom, cleaning herself—all were almost infinitely more difficult for her. Somehow, asking her how she was doing seemed hollow and trite. What a preposterous notion it was that I could even begin to understand how she was doing!

I stepped out of the room and spoke briefly with my supervising resident: The patient had some acute issues and she was having ongoing difficulty after having lost her legs, I explained.

The resident and I went in together and I watched the resident do a nuanced, skilled history and physical exam. We delved more directly into the topic of this woman's emotional state after her surgery. How was she doing at home? How was she coping? What were her moods and how did she feel from day to day? I stood there as the patient explained that she was having a hard time, but was exploring ways to improve her situation. This was a woman who was not giving up or backing down. She had been attending a job-training program for disabled people. As she talked it became clear that this was no matter of dollars and cents. This went to the core of her feeling like a worthwhile human being. She was talking about proving to herself that she had something left to contribute, could be of some use in the world.

But her attempts so far had largely met with failure. She had been having an exceptionally difficult time adapting to the bulky chair and found it overwhelming to think that she could ever be employed, given her physical disabilities. She had spent months in training only to be wrenched away from her aspirations time and time again with the monumental challenges of daily life. Her struggle and her bitterness were palpable as she talked. Every one of her attempts at self-betterment involved overcoming a mountain of doubt, fear, hopelessness. At one point when she was talking about the relative absurdity of ever being employed, she bitterly stated, "I've thought about being a whore but I couldn't even do that. No one would pay." Her frustration barely covered a mountain of raw sadness.

When she suggested she would be useless even as a whore, an awkward silence fell across the room. The bitterness, the pain, the self-loathing had been put into words. In my naïveté, I let her emotions overwhelm me, though I was able to hide it. The resident told the patient she shouldn't say things like that about herself, but it was a limp response. "Am I making you uncomfortable, doctor?" the patient said. Of course she was, but it didn't need to be said.

We stepped out of the room and grabbed the attending physician, a kind, generous woman who worked tirelessly and selflessly for the underserved. She was toward the end of her career, with a sizable belly herself, and she politely listened as we "presented" the patient and then all three of us went back to talk to the patient. By that time, the woman had regained her sense of calm and confidence. The attending broached the topic of things she could do to improve her situation. The patient had a few more questions about that, and then she brought up a topic that comes up all the time. "What should I be eating, doctor? I'm really trying everything I can to lose weight, but it doesn't seem to be helping." The doctor told her to watch out for sugars, to avoid bagels, to use low-fat dairy products, that fat-free milk and reduced-fat cream cheese were in fact very tasty once you got used to them. She did this with considerable enthusiasm and compassion, perhaps hoping that helping her focus on avoiding bagels might take her mind off the inevitable progression of her advanced disease.

I cringed inside. Coming off a 4-year project coauthoring *The China Study,* having spent countless hours reviewing nutrition literature, I knew a major opportunity had just been missed.

I have never forgotten that patient, perhaps because it was one of the first moments when I felt in a visceral way how poorly the medical system can function. Here was a woman who had a problem caused by the simple choices she made every day, but she still seemed unclear about why she was sick or how her choices were impacting her health. At some point years earlier, she had developed diabetes and started visiting doctors. She undoubtedly interacted with compassionate, intelligent physicians, like the attending one that day, who had provided her with the latest diabetes care, including pills and insulin, and yet her disease had progressed. She moved on to a variety of specialists and a surgical team so skilled that they could cut off both legs and not have a single complication result. And yet her disease progressed. She had reaped the rewards of the technological advances that devised an electric wheelchair that would have been unfathomable 50 years ago. And yet her disease progressed. Through all of this, she still was unclear about the dietary advice that could save her life, her legs, her eyes, her kidneys. She had been in the medical system for years and yet her preventable, perhaps even curable, disease had progressed.

As I sat in the tiny, crowded room looking at the stumps just below her knees, bathed in the awkwardness of an inexperienced trainee, I felt to my core the tragedy of this woman who was still asking what she should be eating. The medical system, the dozens of compassionate, intelligent, skilled doctors, nurses, and other professionals she had known had profoundly failed her. We had failed her. She sat there with us that day revealing her raw emotions, her bitterness and lack of self-worth, her pain and difficulty, her disability, and it didn't have to be this way. She was at the end, desperately struggling to improve the future against all the odds, and it didn't have to be this way. If she had changed the food she ate every day years before, this whole process could have been averted.

What she was eating, what you eat, what I eat, has a profound affect on our health. It is more powerful than anything your doctor can give you or do to you.

I tell my patients that the lifestyles choices they make are more important and more powerful for long-term health and disease than any pill or procedure they can get from me or any other doctor. You have learned about a small sample of the evidence that supports a whole-food, plant-based diet for a variety of health outcomes. You have seen the science behind some of the confusing details and hotly contested questions related to the optimal diet. We certainly do not have all the answers in nutrition, and never will. The details and the recommendations will evolve, as they always have. But the message in this book and the weight of evidence supporting it are as strong as they ever need to be for everyone to take action and change their eating and their health, whether they have disease or are hoping to prevent it.

As a physician, and simply as an adult, I am beginning to appreciate that life is fleeting. No matter how hard we grip the reins, we cannot ultimately control what happens or where we end up. I wonder sometimes if this realization is part of gaining some bit of wisdom as I grow older. Like you, I carry with me many experiences shaping my views, like the conversation with the diabetic woman in the wheelchair and many others. So many reinforce to me that diet and lifestyle are so important. They will give you the best chances to avoid some of our most common, unnecessary tragedies. But beyond the long-term benefits, I hope that whatever diet you choose helps you—*right now*—to have a better life, one filled with more connections, more love, more functioning, and more health.

Never before have we had such a deep and broad range of evidence supporting a whole-food, plant-based diet. Never before have we, as a society, had such a need to promote better lifestyles and optimal nutrition. Never before has our planet, through resource depletion and global warming, needed this shift in diet as much as it does today. Never before has a whole-food, plant-based diet been so easy to implement. Never before has it been so tasty, so convenient, so cheap, and so fulfilling.

You now have the tools to make this your life, to give yourself the best odds for your healthiest present and future, and to do it without anxiety or fear. Be well and good luck.

BREAKFAST

QUICK STOVE-TOP OATMEAL

ERIN CAMPBELL

Preparation Time: 10 minutes

This delicious morning staple can be altered daily if you add different toppings. It is a hearty source of long-lasting energy.

2 cups water

½ cup raisins

1 cup old-fashioned (rolled) oats

Optional add-ins:

Chopped fresh fruit or berries of your choice

Ground flaxseed

Nondairy milk

In a medium saucepan, bring the water and raisins to a boil, then add the oats. Lower the heat to medium low.

Allow the oatmeal to cook for 3 to 5 minutes, or until the oats have absorbed much of the water and softened.

Remove from the heat and serve with berries, flaxseed, and milk.

TIP: • Prepare single-serving oatmeal by halving this recipe or following the microwave directions on your package of oats.

MAKES 2 SERVINGS

SLOW-COOKER OATMEAL

ERIN CAMPBELL

Preparation Time: 10 minutes • Slow-Cooker Time: 7 to 9 hours

Hot, creamy oatmeal without the morning preparation time! Prepare at night and let the slow cooker do its work while you sleep.

½ cup steel-cut oats

2 cups water or nondairy milk of your choice

Optional add-ins:

½ cup raisins

½ teaspoon ground cinnamon

1 cup fresh or frozen berries or other chopped fruit

Ground flaxseed

Nondairy milk

In a 1½- to 2-quart slow cooker, combine the steel-cut oats, liquid, and raisins and cinnamon, if using. Fruit can be added at this stage if you want it cooked into your oatmeal or at the end if you prefer fresh fruit as a topping. Cook on low for 7 to 9 hours.

Serve the oatmeal topped with ground flaxseed, fruit, and nondairy milk.

TIPS: • Make a larger number of servings of oatmeal by adding ¼ cup steel-cut oats and 1 cup water for each additional serving.

• If you're making more than 2 to 3 servings at a time, use a larger slow cooker.

MAKES 2 SERVINGS

Tofu Scramble

ERIN CAMPBELL

Preparation Time: 20 minutes

A good tofu scramble recipe allows room for adaptation. It can be made simple or substantial with the addition of beans, greens, and other leftovers. A favorite seasoning blend is important; use more seasoning if you use extra ingredients, which I call add-ins. I make my all-time favorite variation with Southwestern seasoning, greens, and black beans. Serve with toast and fruit.

A few words on pressing tofu: Pressing tofu removes some of its moisture, which is desirable for a dish like scrambled tofu. Drain the liquid from the tofu package. Remove the tofu from the package and wrap it in either a clean dishcloth or several layers of paper towels. Place the wrapped tofu between 2 plates and place a bowl or can of food on the top plate. Remove, unwrap, and use after pressing for 5 to 10 minutes. A longer pressing time makes the tofu firmer and drier. Pressing can be skipped if desired, particularly if using extra-firm tofu, but cooking time may be slightly longer, as the tofu will be wetter.

2 to 3 tablespoons water

1 medium onion, chopped

3 cloves garlic, minced

1 pound firm or extra-firm tofu, drained and pressed

1 teaspoon ground cumin

1/2 teaspoon paprika

1/2 teaspoon ground turmeric

2 teaspoons white miso mixed into 1/4 cup hot water

Juice of 1/2 lemon or 2 tablespoons lemon juice

1/4 cup nutritional yeast

Pinch of black salt (optional—adds an egg-like flavor)

Salt and black pepper to taste

Optional add-ins:

1/2 to 1 teaspoon Arizona Dreaming salt-free Penzeys Spices seasoning blend

1 can (15 ounces) beans of your choice, drained and rinsed

1 cup cooked brown rice or frozen oil-free shredded potatoes, thawed

2 cups chopped fresh spinach

1/4 to 1/2 cup chopped fresh cilantro

1 or 2 tomatoes, chopped

Salsa, to serve

Heat a large nonstick skillet to medium high. Add the water, onion, and garlic. Cook for 3 minutes, or until the onion is translucent, adding more water as necessary to keep the mixture from sticking.

Using your hands, crumble the pressed tofu into the pan. Add the cumin, paprika, and turmeric. Stir together, using a spatula to break up any very large pieces of tofu. Reduce the heat to medium.

Add the miso and water mix, lemon juice, nutritional yeast, and black salt. Mix to combine. Cook until the liquids have evaporated, about 10 minutes.

Add any add-ins you might be using and cook until heated through. Add water as needed to prevent sticking.

Season to taste with salt and pepper.

MAKES 2 TO 4 SERVINGS

Dr. Campbell's Muesli

THOMAS CAMPBELL

Preparation Time: 10 minutes

Top these hearty oats with nondairy milk, fruit, and ground flaxseed to fuel your morning. A few minutes preparing this muesli will yield many, many breakfasts. Have a large, airtight container ready to store the muesli.

42 ounces old-fashioned (rolled) oats

1/4 cup chopped walnuts

1/4 cup sliced almonds

1/4 cup chopped dates

1 cup raisins

Combine all ingredients in a very large bowl or the large container in which you will be storing the muesli.

Store in an airtight container for up to 2 months.

MAKES APPROXIMATELY 30 1/2-CUP SERVINGS

The BEST Banana Bread

ANN ESSELSTYN • *PREVENT AND REVERSE HEART DISEASE,*
BY CALDWELL B. ESSELSTYN JR., MD

Preparation Time: 10 minutes • Baking Time: 1 hour 10 minutes

We usually make this moist and flavorful bread with whole wheat pastry flour. We use a silicone loaf pan for fully oil-free baking.

"This is especially good toasted. Use all whole wheat flour or all barley or spelt flour if you choose. If you do not have heart disease, add ½ cup chopped walnuts or ¼ cup raisins and ¼ cup walnuts."—*Dr. Esselstyn*

1¼ cups whole wheat flour

1 cup barley or spelt flour

1 teaspoon baking powder

1 teaspoon baking soda

1 teaspoon ground cinnamon

3 small ripe bananas or 2 large

1 jar baby-food prunes or ½ cup applesauce

⅓ cup (or less) maple syrup, honey, or sugar

1 egg replacer (1 tablespoon ground flaxseed meal mixed with 3 tablespoons water OR 1½ teaspoons Ener-G egg replacer mixed with 2 tablespoons water)

½ cup raisins

2 teaspoons vanilla extract

¾ cup oat, almond, or fat-free soy milk

1 tablespoon lemon juice

Preheat the oven to 350°F.

In a large bowl, combine the flours, baking powder, baking soda, and cinnamon.

In a medium bowl, mash the bananas. Combine the remaining ingredients with the bananas.

Add the liquid mixture to the flour mixture and stir together gently. Pour the batter into a 9" x 5" loaf pan and bake for 70 minutes, or until a toothpick comes out clean.

MAKES 1 LOAF

CARDAMOM-RAISIN RICE PUDDING

CATHY FISHER • STRAIGHTUPFOOD.COM

Preparation Time: 1 hour 10 minutes, including rice cooking

Rice pudding for breakfast? When rice pudding is made with whole grains and nondairy milk and is minimally sweetened, why not? Shorten the cooking time by making the rice ahead of time or using 2 cups of leftover cooked brown rice.

1 cup brown rice (short, long, basmati, or jasmine)

2 cups water

1/2 teaspoon ground cardamom

1 teaspoon ground cinnamon

1/2 cup raisins

1/3 cup chopped almonds (optional)

2 cups nondairy milk

4 dates, pitted

1 teaspoon vanilla extract (or seeds from 1 vanilla bean)

Additional chopped or sliced almonds for garnish (optional)

In a large pot, combine the rice and water and bring to a boil. Reduce to a simmer, cover, and cook for 45 to 50 minutes (per your type of rice). Remove from the heat and let stand for 10 minutes, covered.

While the rice is cooking, in a bowl, combine the cardamom, cinnamon, raisins, and almonds (if using). In a blender or Vitamix, combine the milk, dates, and vanilla.

Add the wet mixture to the bowl of dry ingredients and combine. Add this to the pot of cooked brown rice, stir thoroughly, and cook on medium low for 10 minutes to incorporate the flavors.

Serve warm or cold in small dessert dishes. Garnish with a sprinkling of chopped or sliced almonds (if using).

TIPS: • Any kind of nondairy milk will work. I like to use soy milk because it is richer and creamier than rice or almond.

• Make sure you get all the pits out of the dates, as they are quite hard when bitten.

• Add fewer dates if you want the pudding to be less sweet.

MAKES 4 TO 6 SERVINGS

PANANA CAKES

LEANNE CAMPBELL • *THE CHINA STUDY COOKBOOK*

Preparation Time: 25 minutes

This is a breakfast for nonbelievers. They won't even know they're getting healthy.

2 cups whole wheat pastry flour	1 cup water
1 teaspoon baking soda	1 cup nondairy milk
1 teaspoon baking powder	2 egg replacers (2 tablespoons ground flaxseed meal mixed with 6 tablespoons water)
½ teaspoon sea salt	
1 teaspoon ground cinnamon	2 tablespoons maple syrup
1 banana, mashed	

In a medium mixing bowl, combine the flour, baking soda, baking powder, sea salt, and cinnamon.

In a separate bowl, combine the mashed banana, water, milk, egg replacers, and maple syrup.

Combine the wet and dry ingredients and stir just enough to remove any lumps. The batter should be pourable. If it seems too thick, add more milk.

Preheat a nonstick skillet or griddle.

Using a ¼-cup measure, pour small amounts of batter onto the heated surface and cook until the top bubbles. Turn with a spatula and cook the second side until golden brown. Serve immediately.

TIPS: • Preheat the pan or griddle so that sprinkles of water dance on it, but not so hot that it smokes.

• Keep the cakes small. They'll be easier to turn.

• Serve with fresh fruit, fruit preserves, applesauce, or syrup.

MAKES 1 DOZEN PANCAKES

BERRY SAUCE

ERIN CAMPBELL

Preparation Time: 10 minutes

This simple sauce takes advantage of the natural sweetness of fruit to create a tasty topping for pancakes, French toast, or even dessert.

½ cup water

4 cups fresh or frozen cherries or berries of your choice, chopped if large

2 tablespoons cornstarch mixed with ¼ cup water

Lemon juice and sweetener of your choice

In a medium nonstick saucepan, combine the water and cherries or berries. Cover and bring to medium heat. Allow the fruit to heat until hot throughout—frozen fruit will take a little longer.

Uncover and reduce the heat to low. Add the cornstarch and water mixture and stir to combine. Cook while stirring frequently for an additional 2 to 5 minutes at medium heat, or until the mixture thickens.

Adjust the thickness of the mixture by adding 1 tablespoon water at a time until you are happy with the consistency.

Adjust the tartness and sweetness to taste using lemon juice and/or a minimal amount of sweetener (maple syrup, agave, and sugar all work well).

MAKES 4 SERVINGS

Potato Scramble

CATHY FISHER • STRAIGHTUPFOOD.COM

Preparation/Stove-Top Cooking Time: 45 minutes • Baking Time: 30 minutes

This recipe is flavorful and hearty. It makes a generous quantity.

2 pounds Yukon gold potatoes (4 or 5 medium)

1 medium yellow onion, chopped

1 medium red bell pepper, chopped

2 cups sliced mushrooms

1 teaspoon dried oregano

1 teaspoon dried basil

$1\frac{1}{2}$ teaspoons granulated garlic

1 teaspoon paprika

1 can (15 ounces) cooked navy beans or other white beans (about $1\frac{1}{2}$ cups)

1 cup chopped tomatoes

4 medium-large collard green leaves, cut into $\frac{1}{2}$-inch pieces (about $1\frac{1}{2}$ cups)

Preheat the oven to 400°F. Line 2 baking sheets with parchment paper. Cut the potatoes, with skin on, into $\frac{1}{2}$-inch cubes. Spread the cubes out evenly on the baking sheets. Bake for 15 minutes. Remove from the oven and, using a spatula, flip the potatoes (this does not have to be precise). Return to the oven and bake for 15 more minutes, or until tender.

In a large skillet over high heat, place 1 tablespoon water. When the water starts to sizzle, add the onion, bell pepper, and mushrooms and cook, stirring frequently, for 3 minutes. Stir in the oregano, basil, garlic, and paprika, adding water as needed.

Decrease the heat to medium and stir in the beans, tomatoes, and collard greens. Cover the pan and cook for 5 more minutes, or until the collards have wilted, stirring once or twice and adding water as needed to prevent sticking. Stir in the cooked potatoes. Serve immediately with ketchup or salsa.

MAKES 4 TO 6 SERVINGS (8 CUPS)

Citrus-Infused French Toast

ERIN CAMPBELL

Preparation Time: 30 minutes

The chickpea flour in this dish contributes a mild, egg-like flavor reminiscent of French toast made with eggs. This flour can be found in the gluten-free baking section of your grocery store as well as in Indian grocery stores as besan flour. Use ¼ cup whole wheat flour instead of chickpea flour if it proves difficult to find.

½ ripe banana

1 cup nondairy milk

Zest of 1 orange or tangerine

Juice of 1 orange or tangerine (¼ to ⅓ cup)

¼ cup chickpea flour

½ teaspoon ground cinnamon

Dash of ground nutmeg

Dash of salt

8 slices whole wheat bread

Optional toppings:

Berry Sauce (page 205)

Fresh fruit

Applesauce

Maple syrup

In a medium bowl, mash the ripe banana until smooth and combine it with all the other ingredients except the bread. Alternatively, blend all the ingredients except the bread in a blender or food processor.

Heat a large, nonstick skillet or griddle to medium high. If you do not have non-stick, use a spray oil and wipe most of it off before heating.

Dip the bread 1 slice at a time into the coating mixture. Coat both sides. Immediately place it on the hot skillet or griddle. Cook for 2 to 3 minutes on each side, or until golden brown.

Repeat this cooking process with the remaining 7 slices of bread.

Serve hot, topped with your choice of Berry Sauce (page 205), fresh fruit, applesauce, or maple syrup.

MAKES 8 SLICES

LUNCH

TASTY TOSTADOS

LEANNE CAMPBELL • *THE CHINA STUDY COOKBOOK*

Preparation Time: 15 minutes

These tostados leave plenty of room for creativity when it comes to toppings. If you can't find whole grain, oil-free, gordita-style tortillas, create a thicker base for this dish by stacking 2 thin tortillas.

1 can (15 ounces) pinto beans, rinsed and drained

4 thick gordita-style tortillas, heated

½ cup finely grated cabbage

1 avocado, diced

½ cup low-sodium salsa (you pick the heat)

In a food processor, blend the pinto beans until smooth.

In a skillet, heat the beans on medium heat for 5 to 6 minutes.

In an ungreased skillet, heat a tortilla over medium heat until it is warm and soft. Spread the bean mixture over the tortilla. Top with cabbage, avocado, and salsa. Repeat with the rest of the tortillas.

TIPS: • Be sure to select a tortilla made without lard.

• Fat-free refried beans can be used in place of pinto beans.

• Top with fresh cilantro if desired.

• Additional toppings that go well with this dish are chopped onions, fresh tomatoes, and olives.

MAKES 4 SERVINGS

QUICK BURGERS

LINDSAY NIXON • *EVERYDAY HAPPY HERBIVORE*

Preparation Time: 5 minutes • Baking Time: 15 minutes

Despite how strikingly simple and fast these burgers are, they are so much better than the low-fat, frozen premade ones! Take the extra 15 minutes to make something you'll be excited to eat. If you don't have instant oats, pulse old-fashioned (rolled) oats a couple times in a food processor to achieve a finer texture.

"I developed these burgers in a hotel room: They're quick, easy, and require very few ingredients. (In fact, except for the beans and a seasoning packet, I sourced all the ingredients from the complimentary 'breakfast bar.') I make these burgers anytime I need a superfast meal or I'm really low on ingredients."—*Lindsay Nixon*

1 can (15 ounces) black beans, drained and rinsed

2 tablespoons ketchup

1 tablespoon yellow mustard

1 teaspoon garlic powder

1 teaspoon onion power

$\frac{1}{3}$ cup instant oats

Preheat the oven to 400°F. Grease a baking sheet or line it with parchment paper and set it aside.

In a mixing bowl, mash the black beans with a fork until mostly pureed but some half beans and bean parts are still left.

Stir in the condiments and spices until well combined. Then mix in the oats.

Divide into 4 equal portions and shape into thin patties.

Bake for 7 minutes, carefully flip over, and bake for another 7 minutes, or until crusty on the outside. Slap onto a bun with extra condiments and eat!

MAKES 4 BURGERS

Zucchini Pritti-Hummus Wrap

CHEF DEL SROUFE • *CHEF DEL'S BETTER THAN VEGAN*

Preparation Time: 25 minutes

Hummus wraps and sandwiches are easy and tasty and can be made with different ingredients. This recipe showcases a filling that complements hummus.

3 large zucchini, sliced ½" thick	Sea salt and black pepper to taste
2 medium yellow onions, diced and divided	2 cups Traditional Low-Fat Hummus (below)
Sea salt and black pepper to taste	4 whole wheat tortillas (10" or 12")
1 medium green bell pepper, diced	4 green onions, thinly sliced
1 medium tomato, diced	

In a medium saucepan over medium-high heat, sauté the zucchini and half of the onions for 6 to 7 minutes, or until the onions start to turn translucent and the zucchini starts to brown. Add water 1 to 2 tablespoons at a time to keep the vegetables from sticking. Season the vegetables with salt and pepper and remove from the pan. Set them aside.

In the same saucepan, sauté the remaining onions and the bell pepper over medium-high heat for 5 minutes. Add the tomato and cook for 5 more minutes. Season with salt and pepper and pour over the zucchini.

To make the wraps, divide the hummus evenly among the tortillas and spoon the vegetables over the hummus. Sprinkle with the green onions and roll up each tortilla.

MAKES 4 LARGE WRAPS

Traditional Low-Fat Hummus

CHEF DEL SROUFE • *CHEF DEL'S BETTER THAN VEGAN*

Preparation Time: 15 minutes

This hummus is rich in flavor without being rich in fat. One 15-ounce can of beans, drained and rinsed, can be used in this recipe. Put tomato slices, lettuce or baby spinach, sliced cucumber, shredded carrots, and hummus on whole grain bread for an impressive and delicious sandwich.

2 cups cooked garbanzo beans, warmed	3 tablespoons lemon juice
6 cloves garlic or to taste	3/4 teaspoon ground cumin
	Sea salt to taste

Combine all ingredients in a food processor and puree until smooth and creamy. Add water if needed to make a smooth consistency.

MAKES 4 SERVINGS

Easy Pasta Salad

ERIN CAMPBELL

Preparation Time: 20 minutes

This is good to take to barbecues or potlucks so you have something wholesome to eat. It is filling, familiar, and tasty, and no one notices the absent oil. It is also kid-friendly. If you buy a fat-free dressing from the store, be careful to choose a low-sugar variety.

16 ounces 100% whole wheat or brown rice pasta	1 can (15 ounces) kidney beans, drained and rinsed
2 large tomatoes, diced	1 can (15 ounces) chickpeas, drained and rinsed
1 red or green bell pepper, seeded and diced	1/4 to 1/2 cup sliced or whole black olives (optional)
1/2 medium to large red onion, diced	
1 crown of broccoli, cut into florets and lightly steamed	1 cup or more of your favorite fat-free, low-sodium salad dressing
	Salt and black pepper to taste

Cook the pasta according to package instructions, drain, rinse with cold water, and place in a large bowl. Add the tomatoes, bell pepper, onion, steamed broccoli, kidney beans, chickpeas, and olives (if using). Mix to combine.

Pour the salad dressing a little at a time over the pasta and vegetable mixture. Stir to combine. Continue adding salad dressing and stirring until the salad is well coated. Season with salt and pepper to taste. Eat at room temperature.

TIP: • Broccoli florets can be lightly cooked with the pasta if added to the pasta pot for the last 2 to 3 minutes of cooking. Drain and rinse with the pasta.

MAKES 4 MAIN ENTRÉES OR 8 SIDE SERVINGS

SIMPLE CHOPPED SALAD

SUSAN VOISIN • FATFREEVEGAN.COM

Preparation Time: 20 minutes

"You can use any vegetable you like raw instead of these—broccoli, cauliflower, snow peas, etc., would all be good. Just chop them all about the same size. You can prepare the veggies in advance, but keep the lettuce separate from any watery ones, such as tomatoes, and assemble the salad just before serving."—*Susan Voisin*

1 heart of romaine

1 cup diced carrots

1 cup halved grape tomatoes

³/₄ cup diced radishes

³/₄ cup diced yellow or red bell peppers

³/₄ cup diced cucumber (about ¹/₂ large)

¹/₂ cup cooked chickpeas

2 tablespoons chopped kalamata olives (optional)

2 tablespoons Fat-Free Balsamic-Raisin Vinaigrette (opposite page) or other fat-free vinaigrette (or more or less to taste)

1 tablespoon Vegan Mayo (page 214)

Freshly ground black pepper to taste

1 tablespoon chopped walnuts (optional)

Leaving the base attached, cut the romaine heart lengthwise three times; rotate it a quarter of a turn and make 2 or 3 more cuts. Then slice it from top to base to make small, bite-size pieces. Wash it in a strainer or salad spinner and then spin well to dry.

Place the romaine into a large bowl and add the other vegetables, chickpeas, and olives (if using). Add the vinaigrette and mayo to taste, being careful not to add too much, as well as a generous grating of black pepper, and toss to combine. Sprinkle with walnuts (if using).

4 GENEROUS SIDE SALADS OR 2 DINNER SALADS

Fat-Free Balsamic-Raisin Vinaigrette

SUSAN VOISIN • FATFREEVEGAN.COM

Preparation Time: 10 minutes

Dressings are one of the hardest foods to adapt, as most people are used to oil or cream bases. This oil-free dressing is a flavorful mix of sweet and tart without the guilt.

½ cup white balsamic vinegar

½ cup water

¼ cup golden raisins (see Tip)

1 large clove garlic

1 teaspoon dried basil

1 teaspoon dried oregano

2 tablespoons Meyer lemon juice or 1 tablespoon regular lemon juice

2 teaspoons chia seeds

1 teaspoon mellow white miso or salt to taste

In a blender, combine all the ingredients and process on high speed until liquefied. Pour into a storage container and refrigerate until thickened slightly. Stir or shake well before using.

TIP: • If you're not using a high-powered blender such as the Vitamix, you may get smoother results by soaking the raisins in the water until they are plump and then blending.

MAKES 12 SERVINGS

Cucumber-Avocado Vinaigrette

CATHY FISHER • STRAIGHTUPFOOD.COM

Preparation Time: 10 minutes

This is a creamy, eye-catching, fresh-flavored dressing.

½ cup diced cucumber, peeled (about ½ of a medium cucumber or 3 ounces)

¼ of an avocado (1 ounce)

¼ cup water

1½ tablespoons brown rice vinegar

1 tablespoon chopped fresh parsley (any type)

1 tablespoon chopped shallot

1 teaspoon Dijon or stone-ground mustard

⅛ teaspoon black pepper

Using a high-speed or standard blender, blend all ingredients until smooth (or to your desired consistency).

MAKES 1 CUP

OCEAN CHICKPEA SANDWICHES

LEANNE CAMPBELL • *THE CHINA STUDY COOKBOOK*

Preparation Time: 10 minutes

Mock tuna salads are a favorite in plant-based cookbooks, and for good reason— these salads are tasty, filling, and familiar. You might want to make a double batch to enjoy throughout the week. Use the Vegan Mayo following this recipe.

1 can (15 ounces) chickpeas, drained and rinsed

5 tablespoons Vegan Mayo (below)

1 tablespoon mustard

4 tablespoons diced dill pickle

4 tablespoons finely diced onion

1 celery stalk, diced

2 tablespoons rice vinegar

1/2 teaspoon kelp powder

Sea salt and black pepper to taste

8 slices whole wheat bread

4 leaves lettuce

4 slices tomato

Place the chickpeas in a food processor and pulse 2 times to roughly chop. Move the chopped chickpeas to a medium-large bowl and add the mayonnaise, mustard, pickle, onion, celery, rice vinegar, kelp powder, salt, and pepper. Mix thoroughly.

Spread the mixture on the bread and top with lettuce and tomato slices.

TIP: • Kelp powder is found in health food stores and adds a great "seafood" taste to this dish.

MAKES 4 SANDWICHES

VEGAN MAYO

LINDSAY NIXON • *EVERYDAY HAPPY HERBIVORE*

Preparation Time: 5 minutes

This zesty mayo is tasty on sandwiches and in salads in which mayo is traditionally used. Unlike many plant-based mayonnaises, it is oil and nut free, making it low calorie.

1 package (12 ounces) Mori-Nu or other shelf-stable silken tofu

2 or 3 tablespoons Dijon mustard

2 teaspoons distilled white vinegar

Lemon juice to taste

Agave nectar to taste

In a blender or small food processor, blend the tofu with the mustard and vinegar until smooth and creamy.

Add a few drops of lemon juice and a few drops of agave nectar and blend again. Taste and add more lemon, agave nectar, or mustard as needed or desired. Chill until ready to use.

TIP: • In a pinch, or for soy-free, substitute plain (preferably unsweetened) vegan yogurt for mayo in recipes.

MAKES 1 CUP

HEARTY EVERYTHING SALAD

ERIN CAMPBELL

Preparation Time: 60 minutes, including rice cooking time

This salad is called the Everything Salad because it has everything, including hearty grains and beans. This is not the dainty rabbit salad consisting primarily of leaves that has you hungry in 45 minutes. Make the rice and lentils ahead of time and reheat prior to topping with salad to cut down on prep time.

2 cups brown rice

$\frac{1}{2}$ cup brown lentils, rinsed

$4\frac{1}{2}$ cups water

6 ounces or more fresh baby spinach, washed and ready to use

3 large tomatoes, cut into thin wedges

1 red or green bell pepper, diced

1 large cucumber, sliced thin

1 cup raw green beans, trimmed and cut to bite-size pieces

$\frac{1}{2}$ medium to large red onion, diced

2 medium carrots, grated

1 can (15 ounces) black beans, drained and rinsed

1 can (15 ounces) chickpeas, drained and rinsed

Fat-free, low-sodium salad dressing of your choice (use prepared or see the recipes on pages 213 and 216)

In a large pot, place the rice, lentils, and water and bring to a boil. Reduce the heat to a simmer and cook for 40 to 50 minutes, or until the rice is tender. Cover the cooked rice with a lid and let it stand for 10 minutes before stirring to fluff it. A rice cooker can easily be used for this step of the recipe. Simply add the ingredients and cook according to rice cooker instructions.

In a large salad bowl, toss the spinach, tomatoes, bell pepper, cucumber, green beans, onion, carrots, black beans, and chickpeas to combine.

Top the still-warm rice and lentil mixture with a generous helping of fresh salad. Top each serving with salad dressing.

MAKES 4 SERVINGS

Strawberry Vinaigrette

CATHY FISHER • STRAIGHTUPFOOD.COM

Preparation Time: 10 minutes

Sweet and tart with a touch of pepper, this is great for any salad.

1 cup sliced strawberries (about 7 medium strawberries)

¼ cup water

1 tablespoon apple cider vinegar

1 tablespoon chopped white or yellow onion

1 Medjool date, pitted and chopped (or 2 deglet noor dates)

1 teaspoon chia seeds

⅛ teaspoon black pepper

Using a high-speed or standard blender, blend all ingredients until smooth (or to your desired consistency).

MAKES 1 CUP

Ensalada Azteca

LEANNE CAMPBELL • *THE CHINA STUDY COOKBOOK*

Preparation Time: 25 minutes

Fresh and flavorful, this salad makes a delicious lunch on its own. Diced frozen mangoes can be used if desired. Allow mangoes to thaw at room temperature before adding. If you don't care for mangoes or you want a less sweet dressing, try dressing the salad with rice vinegar, lime juice, ginger, and sea salt to taste.

For the salad:

2 cans (15 ounces each) black beans, drained and rinsed

2 cups cooked quinoa or brown rice

½ cup finely chopped red onion

1 green bell pepper, diced

1 large tomato, diced

1 large avocado, diced

2 cups frozen corn, thawed

½ cup diced mangoes

1 jalapeño, finely diced

¾ cup chopped fresh cilantro

For the dressing:

1/3 cup unseasoned rice vinegar

2 tablespoons lime juice

1/2 cup diced mangoes

1/4 cup agave nectar

1/2 teaspoon grated ginger

Sea salt to taste

In a large salad bowl, combine the beans, quinoa or rice, onion, pepper, tomato, avocado, corn, mangoes, jalapeño, and cilantro.

In a food processor, place the vinegar, lime juice, mangoes, agave, and ginger. Process until smooth.

Pour the dressing over the salad. Toss gently to mix. Season with salt.

TIP: • Seasoned rice vinegar has a mild sweet-sour flavor that makes it a delicious salad dressing by itself or mixed with other ingredients.

MAKES 8 GENEROUS CUPS

Mango-Lime Bean Salad

ANN ESSELSTYN • *PREVENT AND REVERSE HEART DISEASE*,
BY CALDWELL B. ESSELSTYN JR., MD

Preparation Time: 10 minutes

"Everyone loves this, so double or even triple the recipe! It vanishes in a flash and also works as a salsa. It really is our all-time favorite summer salad. The red onion adds a dash of color. The zest (the peel) intensifies the flavor."
—*Ann Esselstyn*

1 mango, peeled and diced

Red or Vidalia onion, diced, to taste (start with 1/2 onion)

1 can (15 ounces) cannellini beans, drained and rinsed

1/2 cup (or more) chopped fresh cilantro

Juice and zest of 1 juicy lime

Baby lettuce or arugula

Combine all ingredients. Serve on a bed of baby lettuce.

MAKES 2 SERVINGS

Baked Tofu

ERIN CAMPBELL

Preparation Time: 15 minutes • Baking Time: 30 minutes

Baked tofu can be a tasty sandwich fixing or addition to a chili or stew. Tofu absorbs the flavors you prepare it with—don't be shy about using a generous amount of seasoning. Premade blends including garam masala, Italian herb blend, curry powder, and Mrs. Dash seasonings all work well. Use your imagination for seasonings; the possibilities are endless.

A few words on pressing tofu: Pressing tofu removes some of its moisture, which is desirable for a dish like baked tofu. Drain the liquid from the tofu package. Remove the tofu from the package and wrap it in either a clean dishcloth or several layers of paper towels. Place the wrapped tofu between 2 plates and place a bowl or can of food on the top plate. Remove, unwrap, and use after pressing for 5 to 10 minutes. A longer pressing time makes the tofu firmer and drier. Pressing can be skipped if desired, particularly if using extra-firm tofu, but cooking time may be slightly longer, as the tofu will be wetter.

1 package (16 ounces) firm or extra-firm tofu, drained and pressed

Seasoning blend of your choice, preferably salt free

Garlic powder

Onion powder

Salt and black pepper

Preheat the oven to 350°F.

Slice the tofu into 8 to 10 slices of approximately the same size.

Place the tofu slices on a large baking sheet that has been covered with parchment paper or a silicone baking mat, or very lightly coated with cooking spray. Leave space between each slice. Season generously on both sides of the slice with seasoning blend, garlic and onion powders, and salt and pepper.

Bake the tofu slices for 15 minutes.

Remove from the oven and use a spatula to flip each slice over. Return to the oven and bake for an additional 15 minutes, or until lightly browned around the edges.

TIP: • If you prefer cubes of tofu, cut the tofu into cubes and toss the cubes to coat with seasonings in a medium bowl. Spread on the prepared baking sheet and bake as you did with the slices, only reducing each baking time from 15 minutes to 10 minutes.

MAKES 3 OR 4 SERVINGS

SWEET POTATO FRIES

ERIN CAMPBELL

Preparation Time: 5 minutes • Baking Time: 30 minutes

Clearly these are not fast-food French fries, but these fries can become your new family standby. They are filling, easy, tasty, and kid-friendly.

4 large sweet potatoes, scrubbed	**Salt, pepper, and cayenne pepper or salt-free seasoning blend**

Preheat the oven to 400°F.

Cut the sweet potatoes with skins on into long, thin fries.

Place the potatoes on a large baking sheet that has been covered with parchment paper or a silicone baking mat, or very lightly coated with cooking spray. Leave space between each fry.

Sprinkle generously with salt, pepper, and seasonings.

Bake for 15 minutes. Remove from the oven and turn the fries with a spatula.

Return the fries to the oven to bake for an additional 15 minutes, or until crisp and lightly browned.

Serve hot with ketchup.

MAKES 4 SERVINGS

BAKED POTATOES

ERIN CAMPBELL

Preparation Time: 5 minutes • Baking Time: 45 to 60 minutes

Oven-baked potatoes aren't necessarily fast, but they are easy and nice to have for recipes later that day or week. Top these with Chili sans Carne (page 226) for Baked Potatoes Topped with Chili. Use either white or sweet potatoes. Sweet potatoes are extremely healthy, and they cook faster.

4 large baking potatoes, scrubbed   **Aluminum foil**

Preheat the oven to 425°F.

Prick each of the clean potatoes with the tines of a fork and wrap in aluminum foil.

Bake for 45 to 60 minutes, or until you can easily stick a fork in one of the potatoes. Sweet potatoes will need about 40 minutes, depending on size.

TIP: • Baked potatoes can be made in the same way without aluminum foil; the skins will, however, be crisper.

MAKES 4 SERVINGS

Soba Peanut Noodles

LINDSAY NIXON • *HAPPY HERBIVORE LIGHT & LEAN*

Preparation Time: 20 minutes

"All the taste you love in creamy peanut noodles but with less calories and fat thanks to a surprise ingredient: vegan yogurt! I call this a 'cheater' recipe because I use a dab of peanut butter, but it's still light compared to most peanut noodle recipes."—*Lindsay Nixon*

For the noodles:

4 ounces buckwheat noodles (or spaghetti)

2 green onions, sliced

Cubed tofu or edamame (optional)

Vegetables, such as broccoli or cucumber (optional)

For the peanut sauce:

2 tablespoons plain vegan yogurt

1 tablespoon smooth peanut butter

1 tablespoon sweet red chili sauce

Few dashes of garlic powder

Few dashes of ground ginger

1 tablespoon rice vinegar

1 to 2 teaspoons low-sodium soy sauce or gluten-free tamari sauce

Asian hot sauce (e.g., Sriracha; optional)

Cook the noodles according to package instructions, rinse under cold water in a colander, and chill in the fridge for a few minutes if you can.

Meanwhile, whisk the peanut sauce ingredients together. Taste, adding more soy sauce as desired.

Toss the noodles with the sauce, then stir in the green onions, tofu or edamame (if using), and vegetables (if using).

TIP: • Despite having "wheat" in the name, buckwheat flour is completely gluten free. Just make sure your noodles are 100% buckwheat if you have an allergy or sensitivity.

MAKES 2 SERVINGS

DINNER

EASY SPINACH AND MUSHROOM LASAGNA
SUSAN VOISIN • FATFREEVEGAN.COM

Preparation Time: 15 minutes • Baking Time: 60 minutes

This lasagna is a favorite at our house. It is delicious, hearty, and familiar and slices nicely into squares that stay together when serving. We top it with nutritional yeast for an oil-free, Parmesan cheese–like topping. We often cover the top with steamed broccoli before pouring on the top layer of tomato sauce for an extra serving of veggies.

½ pound fresh mushrooms, sliced

1 teaspoon chopped garlic

2 tablespoons water

2 jars (24 ounces each) tomato spaghetti sauce

9 regular lasagna noodles, uncooked

Sliced black olives (optional)

For the filling:

1 pound tofu (firm, reduced-fat recommended—not silken!)

10 ounces frozen chopped spinach, thawed and drained

1 teaspoon salt (optional)

2 tablespoons nutritional yeast (adds a cheesy taste)

1½ teaspoons dried oregano

½ teaspoon garlic powder

1 teaspoon dried basil

½ teaspoon crushed rosemary

⅛ teaspoon cayenne pepper

In a large saucepan, sauté the mushrooms and garlic in the water over medium heat until tender. Cover between stirrings to keep them from drying out. Remove from the heat, add the spaghetti sauce, and stir to combine.

In a food processor, place the tofu and thawed spinach and process briefly. Add the remaining filling ingredients to the processor and blend until smooth. (You may do this without a food processor by using a potato masher on the tofu.)

Preheat the oven to 375°F.

Spread half of the sauce in the bottom of a 9" × 12" pan. Place a layer of noodles over the sauce, using 3 dry noodles and leaving a little space in between them. Spread half of the tofu mixture on the noodles (I drop it by spoonfuls and then spread it). Cover with another layer of 3 noodles and then spread the remaining tofu mixture over them. Top with a final layer of noodles and pour the remaining sauce over this.

Cover the dish tightly with foil and bake for 30 minutes. Then remove the foil and bake for another 30 minutes. Remove from the oven and sprinkle with olives (if using). The lasagna will cut better if you allow it to cool for 15 minutes before serving.

TIP: • If you have a soy allergy, you can make this dish soy free by replacing the tofu with one 15-ounce can of white beans that have been drained and rinsed. Combine with the other filling ingredients as you would with tofu.

MAKES 9 SERVINGS

RICE WITH SALSA, BEANS, AND CILANTRO

ANN ESSELSTYN • *PREVENT AND REVERSE HEART DISEASE,*
BY CALDWELL B. ESSELSTYN JR., MD

Preparation Time: 5 minutes

This recipe is fast and delicious. Use leftover rice for the fastest version. If you don't have leftover rice, make whole wheat couscous in less than 10 minutes to use instead.

1 jar (16 ounces) salsa

1 can (15 ounces) black beans, drained and rinsed

Juice of ½ juicy lime or lemon

Cilantro, lots

Leftover rice

Combine the salsa, beans, juice, and cilantro and serve over reheated rice.

MAKES 2 OR 3 SERVINGS

QUICK THREE-BEAN SOUP

LEANNE CAMPBELL • *THE CHINA STUDY COOKBOOK*

Preparation Time: 10 minutes • Cooking Time: 35 minutes

This is one of the easiest meals in this plan. It also is one of the healthiest, utilizing several varieties of legumes that are loaded with fiber, protein, and many other healthy nutrients. Not much chopping is required, and you'll be able to make it with mostly frozen and pantry ingredients. The soup on its own is great, but try serving it over brown rice for a filling one-pot meal. It makes great leftovers, too.

1 medium onion, diced

4 cloves garlic, minced

2 tablespoons vegetable broth

1 can (15 ounces) black beans, rinsed and drained

1 can (15 ounces) red kidney beans, rinsed and drained

1 can (15 ounces) chickpeas, rinsed and drained

1 can (14 ounces) crushed tomatoes, with jalapeños

2 cups frozen mixed vegetables (corn, green beans, and/or carrots)

1 teaspoon smoked paprika

1 teaspoon black pepper

1 heaping teaspoon dried parsley

1 teaspoon dried oregano

In a large soup pot, sauté the onion and garlic in the broth over medium-high heat until the onion is slightly transparent.

Add the remaining ingredients. Cover and cook on medium-low heat for 30 minutes.

TIPS: • For variety, leafy greens like kale or chard and seasonal vegetables like zucchini, carrots, green beans, and corn are especially good in this recipe as a substitution for the frozen vegetables.

• This soup goes well with Fiesta Corn Bread (page 228).

MAKES 4 TO 6 SERVINGS

MINESTRONE SOUP

CATHY FISHER • STRAIGHTUPFOOD.COM

Preparation Time: 25 minutes • Cooking Time: 50 minutes

Fennel adds a wonderful flavor to this dish. Serve with crusty, 100% whole grain bakery bread for a delightful meal.

"Minestrone is known in Italy as 'the big soup,' since it is thick with colorful ingredients. It has no set list of 'must-have' ingredients, but vegetables in tomato broth with beans and pasta is common. In this version, fresh fennel and fennel seeds are added for even more Mediterranean flair."—*Cathy Fisher*

1 bulb fennel, diced (or 3 ribs celery, diced)

1/2 yellow onion, diced

1/2 cup water, divided

4 cloves garlic, minced

1 teaspoon whole fennel seed

1/4 teaspoon red pepper flakes (optional)

6 cups water

1 box (26 ounces) Pomì chopped tomatoes or 2 cans (15 ounces each) diced tomatoes

3 medium Yukon gold potatoes, diced

2 medium carrots, diced

6 medium white or cremini mushrooms, diced

2 medium zucchini, diced

2 cups cooked kidney beans (or one 15-ounce can, drained)

1/2 cup chopped fresh basil or tarragon

1 cup chopped fresh parsley

2 cups cooked whole grain elbow (or other small) pasta (about 1 1/2 cups dry)

In a large soup pot, sauté the fennel and onion in a couple tablespoons of water for about 5 minutes, adding water as needed to prevent sticking, until tender and fragrant. Add the garlic, fennel seed, and red pepper flakes (if using) along with any of the remaining water and sauté for another 2 minutes.

Add the 6 cups water, tomatoes, potatoes, carrots, mushrooms, zucchini, and beans. Stir well and cook on medium-low heat until the potatoes and carrots are tender, about 30 minutes, stirring occasionally.

Add the basil or tarragon and parsley and stir. Add the cooked pasta and simmer on low for 5 to 10 minutes. Serve hot.

MAKES 6 SERVINGS

CHILI SANS CARNE

LINDSAY NIXON • *THE HAPPY HERBIVORE*

Preparation Time: 45 minutes to 1 hour

This recipe is incredibly delicious and hearty. It is familiar for those who like a meaty taste and consistency, and yet it's incredibly healthy. This is well worth the long list of ingredients.

1 small onion, diced

1 can (28 ounces) diced tomatoes with juice

2 tablespoons chili powder or to taste

1 teaspoon ground cumin

1 teaspoon dried oregano

1 teaspoon granulated garlic powder

1 can (15 ounces) kidney beans, drained and rinsed

1 can (15 ounces) pinto beans, drained and rinsed

1 cup frozen yellow corn

1 tablespoon ketchup

1 tablespoon yellow mustard

1 teaspoon pure maple syrup

1 teaspoon mild curry powder

1 tablespoon vegetarian Worcestershire sauce

1½ cups textured vegetable protein or textured soy protein

2 cups (double recipe) No-Beef Broth (opposite page)

Salt and black pepper to taste

Cayenne pepper to taste

Hot sauce to taste

Line a medium pot with a thin layer of water. Add the onion and cook over medium heat until translucent and most of the water has evaporated, about 3 minutes.

Add the tomatoes with their juice, chili powder, cumin, oregano, and garlic powder and bring to a boil. Once it's boiling, reduce the heat to low, cover, and simmer for 30 to 45 minutes, or until the liquid has reduced slightly.

Add the beans, corn, ketchup, mustard, maple syrup, curry, and Worcestershire sauce, stirring to combine. Cover and turn off the heat, but leave on the warm stove.

Meanwhile, prepare the broth. Combine the textured vegetable protein with the broth, then add to the chili, stirring to combine. Set aside uncovered for 10 minutes. Give it a good stir, then add salt and black pepper. Add cayenne pepper or hot sauce if desired.

MAKES 8 SERVINGS

No-Beef Broth

LINDSAY NIXON • *THE HAPPY HERBIVORE*

Preparation Time: 5 minutes

"There are a few commercial mock beef broth bouillon cubes on the market, but I find all of them a little too salty for my taste. This is my DIY version."
—*Lindsay Nixon*

- 1 tablespoon soy sauce
- 1 tablespoon nutritional yeast
- ½ teaspoon vegetarian Worcestershire sauce
- ¼ teaspoon onion powder
- ¼ teaspoon garlic powder
- ¼ teaspoon ground ginger
- ⅛ teaspoon black pepper
- Salt to taste

In a medium saucepan, whisk all the ingredients together with 1 cup water until well combined.

Bring to a boil and simmer for 1 minute.

If you used water and low-sodium soy sauce, you might want to add a little salt.

TIP • If you use this broth in a soup recipe, add a bay leaf during cooking.

MAKES 1 CUP

Fiesta Corn Bread

LEANNE CAMPBELL • *THE CHINA STUDY COOKBOOK*

Preparation Time: 10 minutes • Baking Time: 35 minutes

Moist and flavorful, this bread will fit right in everywhere you would normally eat corn bread.

1 cup cornmeal

1 cup whole wheat pastry flour

1 teaspoon baking powder

1 teaspoon baking soda

$^1/_2$ teaspoon sea salt

$^1/_2$ teaspoon dried tarragon

$^3/_4$ cup corn, fresh off the cob or thawed

$^1/_3$ cup unsweetened applesauce

2 tablespoons maple syrup

1 egg replacer (1 tablespoon ground flaxseed meal mixed with 3 tablespoons water)

$1^1/_3$ cups soy milk

Preheat the oven to 350°F.

In a large bowl, place the cornmeal, flour, baking powder, baking soda, salt, and tarragon and mix well.

Add the corn, applesauce, and maple syrup to the dry ingredients and mix. Add the egg replacer and milk and stir until everything is well mixed.

Pour into a 9″ x 9″ nonstick baking dish.

Bake for 35 minutes, or until the top is firm and a knife inserted in the center comes out clean. Cool before serving.

TIPS: • Serve with beans and cooked kale or other greens.

• If you want a more Italian herb flavor, add 1 teaspoon dried oregano and 1 teaspoon dried basil.

MAKES 9 SERVINGS

STEAMED KALE

ERIN CAMPBELL

Preparation Time: 12 minutes using prewashed kale

This dish is our go-to vegetable side dish. Buying packaged, prewashed, and chopped kale from the produce department can be a wonderful time-saver. Alternatively, buy bunches of fresh kale and rinse, remove thick stems, chop, and store in a salad spinner ready to use.

½ cup water

3 cloves garlic, minced

½ medium onion, chopped

8–10 ounces kale, washed and chopped with large stems removed

Dash of garlic powder

Dash of onion powder

For the Dijon lemon sauce:

1 tablespoon Dijon mustard

2 tablespoons low-sodium soy sauce (or tamari sauce)

Juice of ½ lemon

In a large sauté pan, heat the water over high heat. Add the minced garlic and onion and cook for 2 to 3 minutes, or until fragrant.

Add the kale and more water as needed to prevent the pan from drying out. Cover the pan and reduce the heat to medium. Steam for approximately 8 to 10 minutes, or until the kale is bright to dark green and tender. Add the garlic and onion powders and stir.

For the Dijon lemon sauce, mix the mustard, soy sauce, and lemon juice in a separate bowl and add to the cooked kale, mixing gently.

Alternative toppings include Miraculous Walnut Sauce (page 240) or flavored balsamic vinegars. Serve hot.

TIPS: • If you don't have a large pan, fill your pan, cover, allow the kale to cook down for 1 to 2 minutes, then add additional handfuls of kale. Repeat until you have added all the kale.

• Sprinkle with cayenne pepper for a spicy kick.

• Add diced tomatoes and white beans toward the end of cooking for a heartier dish.

MAKES 2 TO 4 SERVINGS

SAUTÉED BOK CHOY

ERIN CAMPBELL

Preparation Time: 10 minutes

Bok choy is unfamiliar to many people, but it has a wonderful smooth, mild taste that goes well with many different sauces. It packs all the nutrition of a dark leafy green.

¼ cup + 1 tablespoon water

3 cloves garlic, minced

1 teaspoon fresh gingerroot, minced or grated

Pinch of red pepper flakes (optional)

1½ pounds bok choy or baby bok choy, washed, ends cut off, and cut diagonally into pieces

1 tablespoon low-sodium soy sauce

1 tablespoon orange juice

1 teaspoon sesame seeds (optional)

In a large sauté pan, place ¼ cup of the water. Bring the pan to medium-high heat. Add the garlic and ginger and sauté for 2 to 3 minutes, or until fragrant. Add the red pepper flakes (if using).

Add the bok choy to the pan, along with additional water as needed. Cover with a lid and cook at medium for 2 to 3 minutes, or until the bok choy is bright green and tender-crisp.

In a separate bowl, mix the soy sauce, orange juice, and remaining 1 tablespoon water. Add to the greens and mix gently. Garnish with sesame seeds (if using). Serve hot.

TIP: • Peel fresh gingerroot and store it in a container in the freezer. Use a microplane or grater to shred frozen gingerroot as you need it for recipes, placing the remaining gingerroot back in the freezer. Ginger stays fresh and ready to use.

MAKES 4 SERVINGS

GLOBAL GREENS

CATHY FISHER • STRAIGHTUPFOOD.COM

Preparation Time: 15 minutes • Cooking Time: 15 minutes

"I call this dish 'global' because it lends itself to a variety of seasonings—choose your favorite! Kale, chard, Brussels sprouts, yellow onion, white beans, and a sprinkling of whole mustard seeds come together quickly and beautifully all in one pot."—*Cathy Fisher*

1¼ cups water, divided

1 yellow onion, cut into long pieces along the grain

4 cloves fresh garlic, minced

1 tablespoon whole yellow mustard seeds

2 teaspoons Mexican seasoning blend, or another blend of your choice (see Tips)

1 can (15 ounces) cannellini or navy beans, drained and rinsed (1½ cups)

20 Brussels sprouts, ends trimmed, cut in half lengthwise

1 bunch curly kale (6–8 large leaves)

1 bunch chard (4–6 large leaves)

Heat a large skillet or soup pot on high heat with ¼ cup water in the bottom. When the water begins to sizzle and the pan is hot, add the onion and sauté it for 3 to 5 minutes, or until the onion softens and its edges begin to turn light brown. Add a tablespoon or two of water as needed to prevent sticking.

Add the minced garlic, mustard seeds, seasoning, and beans and sauté while mixing for another minute until all the seasoning is incorporated, adding a little water as needed. Add the Brussels sprouts and greens and cover the pot. Turn the heat to medium and cook for 5 to 7 minutes, stirring a few times and checking that there is a thin layer of liquid in the bottom. (By the end of making this dish, all 1¼ cups of water will be used.)

When the Brussels sprouts are tender, stir through a couple times, and the dish is ready to serve. Optional: Top with some pumpkin seeds or pine nuts, whole or grated (with a rotary cheese grater).

TIPS: • Seasoning blends: I used a Mexican seasoning blend made up of chile pepper, onion, paprika, cumin, and oregano. Pretty much any blend will work here, including an "all-purpose" kind. But also consider the following blends: Cajun, Caribbean, Mediterranean, garam masala, curry, Italian, or chili powder. For curry, garam masala, or chili powder blends, you may want to start with 1 teaspoon and then taste, as these are spicier than other types. (A quarter to ½ teaspoon of hot red pepper flakes would also make a nice addition for those who like an extra-spicy kick.)

• Greens: I used curly kale and chard, but you may also use other greens, such as beet or collard greens or Russian or dinosaur kale. I usually trim off the thickest part of the stems and discard them, but you can eat them; they just need to be cooked a little longer than the leaves (wash and dice the stems and add them in with the onions so that they soften).

MAKES 2 TO 4 SERVINGS

Sautéed Baby Spinach

ERIN CAMPBELL

Preparation Time: 7 minutes

Baby spinach has a milder taste than mature spinach. It cooks down substantially, so don't be shy about filling the pan with leaves.

⅓ cup + 1 tablespoon water

4 cloves fresh garlic

9 ounces baby spinach, washed and ready to use

¼ teaspoon onion powder

¼ teaspoon garlic powder

1 tablespoon low-sodium soy sauce (or tamari sauce)

1 tablespoon orange juice

Heat ⅓ cup of the water in a large sauté pan over high heat. Add the garlic and cook for 2 to 3 minutes, or until fragrant.

Add the spinach and more water as needed to prevent the pan from drying out. Cover the pot and reduce the heat to medium. Steam for approximately 3 minutes, or until the spinach is bright to dark green and tender. Add the onion and garlic powders and mix gently.

In a small bowl, combine the soy sauce, orange juice, and remaining 1 tablespoon water and pour over the hot spinach. Serve hot.

TIPS: • Chopped onion and bite-size pieces of baked tofu are tasty additions to steamed spinach.

• Instead of soy sauce, orange juice, and water topping, try flavored balsamic vinegars for variety.

MAKES 2 TO 4 SERVINGS

Rainbow Greens

LINDSAY NIXON • *EVERYDAY HAPPY HERBIVORE*

Preparation Time: 10 minutes

The raisins add a nice sweetness to these slightly bitter but beautiful greens.

1 bunch rainbow chard, well rinsed	1 teaspoon apple cider vinegar
4 cloves garlic, minced	¼ cup raisins
Pinch of dried oregano	Salt and black pepper

Although it is best to remove the stems from most leafy greens, leave them intact here. (If you use collards or kale, you'll want to cut away the stems.) Coarsely chop the chard and set it aside.

Line a large pot or skillet with a thin layer of water.

Add the garlic, oregano, and vinegar and bring to a boil, sautéing the garlic over high heat for 1 minute.

Add the raisins and cook for another minute, then add the chard. Use tongs or a spatula to stir the chard around so it cooks down and incorporates with the other ingredients.

Once the chard is softer and brighter in color, turn off the heat and mix everything well.

Season with salt and pepper.

MAKES 2 SERVINGS

Pineapple Stir-Fry

LINDSAY NIXON • *HAPPY HERBIVORE LIGHT & LEAN*

Preparation Time: 20 minutes

"Quick, easy, and delicious. This light stir-fry doesn't feel like a slimmed-down dish. It's still big on taste without coconut milk. If you'd like to add another vegetable to bulk up the dish, try broccoli. Serve over brown rice or quinoa."—*Lindsay Nixon*

1/2 cup vegetable broth	1 cup pineapple chunks
4 green onions, sliced	1/4 cup pineapple juice
3 cloves garlic, minced	1 cup diced tofu
1 tablespoon minced fresh gingerroot	1 teaspoon cornstarch mixed into 2 tablespoons water
Pinch of red pepper flakes	
1 tablespoon brown rice vinegar	2–3 tablespoons chopped fresh cilantro (optional)
1 tablespoon low-sodium soy sauce or gluten-free tamari sauce	Asian hot sauce (e.g., Sriracha; optional)
1 tablespoon sweet red chili sauce	
1 red bell pepper, seeded and sliced into strips	

Line a skillet with a thin layer of broth. Sauté the white and light green parts of the onions (reserving the dark parts for later), garlic, ginger, and a dash or two of red pepper flakes for a few minutes, until fragrant.

Add the vinegar, soy sauce, chili sauce, bell pepper, and a splash of broth—enough so there is a thin layer of liquid in the skillet. Continue to sauté, adding broth as necessary, until the peppers are tender but still crisp.

Add the pineapple chunks, juice, and tofu and stir to combine.

Add the cornstarch and continue to cook and stir, until the sauce has thickened.

Stir in the cilantro (if using). Garnish with leftover green onion and additional cilantro as desired. Add a drizzle of hot sauce for a spicier dish if desired.

TIP: • Rice vinegar may be substituted for the brown rice vinegar.

MAKES 2 SERVINGS

Burrito Bar

ERIN CAMPBELL

Preparation Time: 20 minutes or less

This meal is more of a meal idea than a true recipe. Buy and prep simple burrito ingredients. There is plenty of room for creativity. The number of servings varies by the number of tortillas and fillings you have on the ready.

Suggestions for burrito ingredients:

Whole, sprouted-grain tortillas (oil free)

Whole grain corn and wheat tortillas (oil free)

Brown rice seasoned with Mexican or Southwest seasoning blend

Black beans, drained and rinsed

Fat-free refried beans

Baby spinach, chopped

Cabbage, shredded

Bell pepper, chopped

Red or sweet onion, chopped

Tomato, diced

Salsa

Cilantro, chopped

Avocado, diced

Baked tofu cubes

In a dry skillet on medium heat or in the microwave, warm the tortillas until soft and hot. In skillets or in the microwave, warm rice, black beans, and refried beans.

Fill each tortilla with your ingredients of choice. Fold in both ends and roll up.

MAKES 2 TO 6 SERVINGS

Dr. Campbell's Bachelor Meal

THOMAS CAMPBELL

Preparation Time: 15 to 20 minutes

No preparation, one pot, minimal cleanup, fast, with leftovers. What more could a bachelor want? The flavors are determined by the prepared soup. This recipe won't win any innovative cooking awards, but it will help you eat something healthier than takeout if you are low on time, energy, or ingredients.

16 ounces 100% whole wheat or brown rice pasta

2 large boxes or cans (17 to 19 ounces each) of an oil-free, plant-based soup

2 cups water (approximately)

9 ounces fresh baby spinach, washed

2 cups (approximately) frozen mixed vegetables of your choice

In a large stockpot, combine all ingredients. Bring to a boil and then lower the heat to a simmer until the pasta is al dente. Add more water to create more of a soup than a pasta, if you prefer.

TIP: • Look for soups with no oil added or soups that are very low in fat. A few good soups for this dish include Pacific Spicy Black Bean & Kale Soup, Dr. McDougall's Lentil All Natural Soup, and Progresso 99% Fat-Free Lentil Soup.

MAKES 4 SERVINGS

Fabulous Sweet Potato Enchiladas

LEANNE CAMPBELL • *THE CHINA STUDY COOKBOOK*

Preparation Time: 20 minutes • Baking Time: 25 minutes

These enchiladas are tasty and filling. The heat in this dish comes from the salsa, so choose your salsa accordingly. If you like your enchiladas saucy, feel free to add more salsa than the one jar the recipe calls for. Use lower-sodium soy sauce to decrease the sodium content (the taste remains delicious).

½ cup vegetable broth, divided

1 medium onion, diced

3 cloves garlic, minced

1 teaspoon ground coriander

1 teaspoon ground cumin

2 cups chopped fresh spinach

2 cups black beans, chopped in food processor or partially mashed by hand

4 tablespoons soy sauce

3 cups cooked, mashed sweet potatoes

Sea salt to taste

10 large tortillas

1 jar of your favorite salsa

Preheat the oven to 350°F.

Heat 2 tablespoons of the vegetable broth. Add the onion and garlic. Sauté until the onion is translucent. Add the coriander and cumin. Cook for 1 minute, stirring constantly.

Add the remaining vegetable broth, spinach, beans, soy sauce, and sweet potatoes. Cook for 3 to 5 minutes. Remove from the heat and season with salt.

Place ¼ to ½ cup of the mixture in the center of a tortilla. Roll into a burrito and place in a nonstick baking dish.

Once all the burritos are assembled, pour your favorite salsa on top and cover with aluminum foil.

Bake for 25 minutes.

MAKES 6 TO 8 SERVINGS

CREAMY PASTA AND BROCCOLI

CHEF DEL SROUFE • *CHEF DEL'S BETTER THAN VEGAN*

Preparation Time: 35 minutes (including Cauliflower Puree)

Unlike creamy vegan pasta recipes made with nuts, this saucy pasta dish tastes great while staying light. It's perfect for people interested in reversing heart disease.

12 ounces whole grain penne pasta	2 tablespoons nutritional yeast
1 head broccoli, cut into florets	2 teaspoons Dijon mustard
2 large leeks, thinly sliced	Zest of 1 lemon
½ cup white wine	Pinch of ground nutmeg
2 cups Cauliflower Puree (opposite page)	Sea salt and black pepper to taste

Cook the pasta according to package instructions. Add the broccoli to the pot of pasta in the last 4 minutes of cooking.

While the pasta and broccoli cook, sauté the leeks in a large skillet until they are tender, about 7 to 8 minutes. Add water 1 to 2 tablespoons at a time to keep the leeks from sticking.

Turn the heat up to high, add the wine, and cook until the liquid is reduced by half. Add the cauliflower puree, yeast, mustard, lemon zest, and nutmeg. Add salt and pepper to taste.

While the sauce is reducing, drain the cooked broccoli and pasta. Before serving, toss with the sauce.

MAKES 4 SERVINGS

Cauliflower Puree

CHEF DEL SROUFE • *CHEF DEL'S BETTER THAN VEGAN*

Preparation Time: 20 minutes or less

"Traditional white sauces are made from cream or milk. Vegan white sauces are usually made from plant milk or silken tofu. My favorite white sauce is made from cauliflower puree. It is one of the most adaptable sauces I make, and much like its dairy-based counterpart, it takes on the flavor of whatever you use to season it."—*Chef Del*

3 cups cauliflower florets

Sea salt to taste

¾ to 1 cup water or vegetable stock

Place the cauliflower in a steamer and cook until very tender, about 8 to 10 minutes.

Place the florets in a blender and puree with enough water or vegetable stock to make a creamy consistency. Season with salt.

TIP: • Use precut cauliflower or frozen cauliflower florets to speed preparation time.

MAKES 2 CUPS

Miraculous Walnut Sauce

ANN ESSELSTYN • *PREVENT AND REVERSE HEART DISEASE,*
BY CALDWELL B. ESSELSTYN JR., MD

Preparation Time: 10 minutes

"Great on greens! Use sparingly, as this sauce is calorie dense. Note: This sauce is not for those with heart disease unless used very sparingly." —*Ann Esselstyn*

½ cup walnuts

1 clove garlic

1–2 tablespoons low-sodium tamari sauce

½ cup (or more) water, depending on how thin or thick you want the sauce

In a blender or food processor, place the walnuts, garlic, and tamari.

Blend, adding as much water as necessary (about ½ cup) to make it the right consistency to pour. It can be quite thin and goes a long way. And it is good on absolutely everything.

MAKES 1 CUP OR MORE

Garden Pizza

ERIN CAMPBELL

Preparation Time: 15 minutes (after crust has been prepared)

Baking Time: 13 minutes

Pizza without cheese? Made with plenty of sauce and toppings, a good cheeseless pizza satisfies without cheese.

Tomato sauce (find a thick, oil-free variety)

2 whole wheat pizza crusts (opposite page)

Mushrooms, sliced

Green pepper, seeded and sliced into thin strips

Broccoli, cut into florets

Red onion, sliced

Cherry tomatoes, halved

Nutritional yeast

Black pepper and Italian herbs

Baby spinach, chopped

Preheat the oven to 425°F.

Spread a thin layer of tomato sauce over the unbaked crusts. Evenly top the pizzas with all vegetables except the spinach.

Top the pizzas with the nutritional yeast, pepper, and Italian herbs.

Bake for 12 to 13 minutes. Top with spinach while still hot.

TIP: • If you can find 100% whole wheat pizza dough or crusts with no added oil, you can use these instead of making a homemade crust. Whole wheat pitas can serve as mini pizza crusts in a pinch.

MAKES 2 TO 4 SERVINGS

Whole Wheat Pizza Dough

CHEF DEL SROUFE • *CHEF DEL'S BETTER THAN VEGAN*

Preparation Time: 1 hour and 20 minutes (including time dough rests and rises)

Wholesome and tasty, these pizza crusts are great with a variety of toppings.

1 envelope active dry baking yeast

1 tablespoon cane sugar

1 cup warm water (about 110°F)

$\frac{1}{2}$ teaspoon sea salt

About 2 cups whole wheat bread flour, divided

In a large bowl, add the yeast and sugar to the warm water and whisk them together. Let the mixture sit until it begins to foam, then add the salt and, using a whisk, stir in 1 cup of the flour. Beat the dough for 75 strokes. Add as much of the remaining flour as needed to make the dough a little stiff but still a little tacky to the touch.

Cover the dough with plastic wrap and let it sit in a warm place until it has doubled in volume, about 45 minutes. Punch it down and let it rise again, about 20 minutes.

Divide the dough into 2 pieces and shape into 2 round, flat crusts. Use in any recipe that calls for whole wheat pizza dough or crust, following the recipe's topping and baking instructions.

MAKES 2 CRUSTS

Cumin-Infused Vegetables and Chickpeas over Quinoa

SUSAN VOISIN • FATFREEVEGAN.COM

Preparation Time: 20 minutes • Cooking Time: 30 minutes

Don't get scared by the longer ingredient list. This recipe uses a variety of spices to make ordinary vegetables richly flavored, even exotic.

½ large onion, chopped

2 cloves garlic, minced

2 teaspoons ground cumin

½ teaspoon ground turmeric

1 teaspoon smoked paprika

¼ teaspoon ground cardamom

⅛ teaspoon cayenne pepper (or more to taste)

2 cups cauliflower florets

½ medium eggplant, cut into ½" cubes

1 can (15 ounces) chickpeas, rinsed and drained

1 can (15 ounces) diced tomatoes (fire-roasted preferred), with juice

½ cup raisins

½ cup water

1 medium zucchini, cut into ½" cubes

¾ cup quinoa, rinsed well and drained

1½ cups vegetable broth (or water with vegetable bouillon or ½ teaspoon salt)

1 clove garlic, minced

Harissa or hot chili sauce for the table

Heat a large nonstick skillet over medium-high heat. Add the onion and sauté for 2 minutes. Sprinkle in the garlic, cumin, turmeric, paprika, cardamom, and cayenne and cook for 2 more minutes, stirring often.

Stir in the cauliflower, eggplant, chickpeas, tomatoes, raisins, and water. Cover the pan and lower the heat to medium. Cook, stirring occasionally, for 10 minutes. Add the zucchini and continue to cook covered until it is just beginning to be tender, about 10 minutes. Add salt to taste.

While the vegetables are cooking, heat a large saucepan and add the quinoa. Toast it, stirring constantly, until it is almost dry. Add the vegetable broth and the garlic, bring to a boil, and stir in the salt if you're using it. Turn the heat to very low, cover, and cook for 15 to 20 minutes, until all liquid is absorbed. Remove from the heat until needed. Fluff with a fork before serving. Serve with the vegetable mixture mounded in the center of the quinoa and a jar of harissa or hot chili sauce for individual seasoning.

MAKES 4 SERVINGS

SLOPPY LENTIL JOES

ANN ESSELSTYN • *PREVENT AND REVERSE HEART DISEASE,*
BY CALDWELL B. ESSELSTYN JR., MD

Preparation Time: 10 minutes • Cooking Time: 60 minutes

Another kid-friendly recipe, this is a tasty, hearty, and easy version of an age-old classic. Don't be shy about using plenty of cilantro, which gives it a wonderful fresh taste.

$3^1/_2$ cups water, divided

1 large onion, chopped (1 cup)

1 bell pepper—any color—seeded and chopped (1 cup)

1 tablespoon chili powder

$1^1/_2$ cups dried lentils, red or brown

1 can (15 ounces) crushed or diced tomatoes

1 tablespoon low-sodium tamari sauce or Bragg Liquid Aminos

2 tablespoons mustard, Dijon or your choice

1 tablespoon brown sugar (optional)

1 tablespoon rice vinegar

1 teaspoon vegetarian Worcestershire sauce

1 bunch cilantro, chopped

Freshly ground black pepper to taste

Place $^1/_3$ cup of the water in a large pot. Add the onion and bell pepper and cook about 5 minutes, or until the onion softens slightly, stirring occasionally.

Add the chili powder and mix well.

Add the remaining water, the lentils, tomatoes, and the rest of the ingredients. Mix well, bring to a boil, lower the heat, cover, and cook over low heat for 55 minutes, stirring occasionally.

MAKES 8 TO 10 SERVINGS

Pumpkin Gnocchi with Italian Vegetable Sauce

LEANNE CAMPBELL • *THE CHINA STUDY COOKBOOK*

Preparation Time: 25 minutes • Cooking Time: 25 to 30 minutes

This is a delicious and satisfying recipe that is surprisingly easy to make. The orange color of the gnocchi in contrast with the red and green of the vegetables is very appealing to the eye.

1 can (15 ounces) pumpkin puree	1 teaspoon dried basil
2¾ cups whole wheat pastry flour	1 tablespoon dried oregano
8 to 10 cups water	1 can (28 ounces) diced tomatoes with jalapeños
1 teaspoon sea salt	
1 medium onion, sliced in long strips	2 large zucchini, sliced
2 tablespoons vegetable broth	Salt and black pepper to taste

Mix the pumpkin and flour to make a soft dough. If necessary, add more flour so the dough holds together and is not sticky. (Be careful not to overwork the dough.)

Divide the dough into 4 or 5 sections and place on a floured surface. Roll each piece into a rope about 1″ in diameter. Cut the rope into 1″ pieces.

In a large pot, add the water and salt. Bring to a boil. Add the gnocchi to the boiling water and cook until the gnocchi rises to the surface and floats, about 5 minutes. Depending on the size of your pot, you may need to cook them in batches. Remove from the water and set aside.

In a large saucepan over medium heat, sauté the onion, vegetable broth, basil, and oregano until the onion is soft, about 4 to 5 minutes. Add the tomatoes and zucchini. Cover and cook for 5 to 7 more minutes, until the zucchini is softened.

Place the vegetables on top of the gnocchi and serve immediately. Season with salt and pepper.

MAKES 6 SERVINGS

DESSERTS

PINEAPPLE SPONGE CAKE

LINDSAY NIXON • *EVERYDAY HAPPY HERBIVORE*

Preparation Time: 10 minutes • Baking Time: 20 minutes

Sweetened only with pineapple chunks and juice, this recipe comes together quickly for what seems like a fancy dessert.

1 can (15 ounces) pineapple rings (in 100% juice)

1 cup whole wheat pastry flour

1 teaspoon baking powder

1 teaspoon baking soda

Pinch of salt

3 dashes of ground ginger

1 teaspoon vanilla extract

Orange zest (optional)

Extra juice for serving

Preheat the oven to 350°F. Grease an 8" or 9" cake pan and set aside.

Drain the pineapple juice into a small bowl and set aside.

In a mixing bowl, whisk the flour, baking powder, baking soda, salt, and a few dashes of ground ginger together. Add the vanilla and zest (if using) and set aside.

Chop the pineapple rings really well or send them through your blender until they have the consistency of crushed, minced pineapple but not puree.

Mix the pineapple into the flour mixture, stirring to combine.

Add the pineapple juice, starting with ¼ cup and then adding a tablespoon at a time, until the batter is just combined and wet, about 6 tablespoons total.

Transfer to a pan and bake for approximately 20 minutes.

Pour the leftover juice, plus additional juice, over the top immediately before serving. You want the cake to be wet and nearly falling apart.

TIP: • Make sure the pineapple rings you buy come in 100% juice and not syrup.

MAKES 9 SERVINGS

FROZEN BANANA CREAM

LEANNE CAMPBELL • *THE CHINA STUDY COOKBOOK*

Preparation Time: 15 minutes

This is a staple dessert in our house. It is smooth, creamy, and sweet—the perfect ending to a healthy meal. If you ever tire of chocolate sauce or want more variety, try topping it with fruit or berry sauce.

For the sauce:

3 tablespoons cocoa powder

3 tablespoons sucanat or packed brown sugar

$\frac{1}{2}$ cup soy milk

For the banana cream:

4 frozen bananas

$\frac{1}{2}$ cup nondairy milk

$\frac{1}{2}$ teaspoon vanilla extract (optional)

In a small saucepan, bring the cocoa, sucanat or brown sugar, and milk to a boil. Reduce the heat and cook until slightly thickened, while stirring constantly. Remove from the heat and set aside.

In a food processor, blend the bananas, milk, and vanilla (if using) until smooth.

Portion the banana mixture into 4 serving bowls. Drizzle the sauce on top of the banana cream and serve immediately.

TIP: • Fresh fruit can be used in place of chocolate topping.

MAKES 2 TO 4 SERVINGS

BANANA-MAPLE OATMEAL COOKIES

SUSAN VOISIN • FATFREEVEGAN.COM

Preparation Time: 15 minutes • Baking Time: 12 minutes

Moist, perfectly sweet, and wholesome, these are some of my favorite cookies to bake for a crowd. They vanish almost instantly, and no one asks if they are healthier than your average cookie. They can also be made with whole wheat pastry flour.

1 teaspoon ground chia seeds or 2 teaspoons egg replacer powder or 2 teaspoons ground flaxseed

2 tablespoons water

1 cup old-fashioned (rolled) or quick oats

1 cup white whole wheat flour

$\frac{1}{2}$ teaspoon baking soda

$\frac{1}{2}$ teaspoon baking powder

$\frac{1}{2}$ teaspoon salt

1 teaspoon cinnamon

$\frac{1}{4}$ cup raisins

$\frac{1}{2}$ teaspoon vanilla extract

½ cup maple syrup	½ teaspoon lemon juice
1 banana, mashed	

Preheat the oven to 375°F.

In a small mixing bowl, combine the chia seeds, egg replacer, or flaxseed with the water and set aside until thickened. No waiting is necessary if packaged egg replacer is used.

In a medium mixing bowl, combine the oats, flour, baking soda, baking powder, salt, and cinnamon. Add the raisins.

Add the vanilla, maple syrup, banana, and lemon juice to the chia/flax/egg replacer mixture and combine well. Pour into the dry mixture and stir well but don't overmix.

Drop by heaping tablespoons onto a baking sheet lined with a silicone mat or parchment paper. Flatten each cookie slightly with a fork. Bake for 8 to 12 minutes, or until the bottoms and sides are lightly brown. Cool for a few minutes on a wire rack before serving.

MAKES 18 COOKIES

CHOCOLATE NO-BAKE COOKIES

KAREN CAMPBELL

Preparation Time: 15 minutes

This is an old Campbell family recipe. It makes for a supereasy, filling, fiber-rich dessert to pack in kids' lunches.

3 tablespoons cocoa powder	¼ cup peanut butter
¼ cup sucanat or packed brown sugar	1 teaspoon vanilla extract
⅓ cup nondairy milk	1 cup old-fashioned (rolled) oats

In a small saucepan, combine all ingredients but the oats. Stir the ingredients together over medium-low heat until combined and the sweetener is dissolved. Remove from the heat.

Add the oats to the mixture in the saucepan, stirring until combined. Allow the cookie dough to cool enough to handle by hand.

Scoop the dough by generous rounded tablespoons into individual cookies. Roll each cookie by hand into a ball.

Cool to room temperature before storing.

MAKES 18 COOKIES

Mixed Fruit Cobbler

LEANNE CAMPBELL • *THE CHINA STUDY COOKBOOK*

Preparation Time: 10 minutes • Baking Time: 25 minutes

Traditional fruit cobbler tops wholesome fruit with an unhealthy mixture of butter and refined flour. This cobbler retains its fruity goodness without those ingredients.

For the filling:

- 4 cups berries; if frozen, thaw first (use blueberries, blackberries, raspberries, or a mixture)
- 3 tablespoons maple syrup

For the crust:

- 1 cup whole wheat pastry flour
- 4 tablespoons sucanat or packed brown sugar
- 1 teaspoon baking powder
- $\frac{1}{2}$ cup almond milk

For the filling, preheat the oven to 400°F.

In a large bowl, combine the berries and maple syrup. Spread in a 9" x 9" baking dish.

In a separate bowl, for the crust, combine the flour, sucanat or brown sugar, and baking powder. Add the milk and stir to mix.

Spread the mixture over the berries (don't worry if they aren't completely covered) and bake until golden brown, about 25 minutes. Let cool for 10 minutes before serving.

MAKES 6 SERVINGS

Chocolate Pudding

ERIN CAMPBELL

Preparation Time: 15 minutes

This pudding is easy, dairy-free, and kid-friendly.

3 tablespoons cornstarch

⅓ cup sucanat or packed brown sugar

⅓ cup cocoa powder

½ teaspoon ground cinnamon

2 cups nondairy milk

1½ teaspoons vanilla extract

Fruit for topping (optional)

In a medium saucepan off the heat, place the cornstarch, sucanat or brown sugar, cocoa powder, and cinnamon. Add the nondairy milk and whisk to combine. The mixture does not need to be thoroughly combined and smooth at this stage. It will continue to combine over the heat.

Heat the saucepan to medium. Bring the mixture to a low boil and stir until it begins to thicken, between 5 and 7 minutes. Turn off the heat once the mixture is thick. Stir in the vanilla. Chill prior to serving if desired.

Top with fruit (if using).

TIPS: • Spices commonly added to sweet desserts—cinnamon, nutmeg, ginger, and cardamom—can be added to desserts to maintain a sweet flavor while reducing the amount of sweetener in the recipe.

• If you prefer a sweeter pudding, add additional sweetener 1 tablespoon at a time prior to heating.

MAKES 4 SERVINGS

AMAZINGLY DELICIOUS DATE FRUIT PIE

LEANNE CAMPBELL • *THE CHINA STUDY COOKBOOK*

Preparation Time: 25 minutes (plus 1 hour chilling time)

This is a truly luxurious dessert in both taste and appearance. Let your artist take over when you arrange the fruit filling and you'll have a truly beautiful dessert. If you want to impress at a dinner party, this is your ticket.

For the crust:

- 1 cup pitted dates
- 1½ cups walnuts (or pecans)
- 1 teaspoon vanilla extract
- ½ cup shredded coconut
- ½ teaspoon cinnamon

For the topping:

- Sliced fresh fruit (½ cup each of strawberries, blackberries, blueberries, mangoes, and kiwis)

In a food processor, blend all crust ingredients at high speed until a paste forms.

Press into a pie pan and chill until ready to add fruit.

Arrange the fruit on top of the crust.

Chill for 1 hour before serving.

MAKES 8 SERVINGS

INTRODUCTION

1. Whitlock EP, Orleans CT, Pender N, and Allan J. Evaluating primary care behavioral counseling interventions: An evidence-based approach. *American Journal of Preventive Medicine* 2002;22:267–284.

CHAPTER 1

1. Youngman LD and Campbell TC. The sustained development of preneoplastic lesions depends on high protein intake. *Nutrition and Cancer* 1992;18:131–142.
2. Schulsinger DA, Root MM, and Campbell TC. Effect of dietary protein quality on development of aflatoxin B1-induced hepatic preneoplastic lesions. *Journal of the National Cancer Institute* 1989;81:1241–1245.
3. Brody J. Huge study of diet indicts fat and meat. *New York Times*, May 8, 1990.
4. Campbell TC and Junshi C. Diet and chronic degenerative diseases: Perspectives from China. *American Journal of Clinical Nutrition* 1994;59:1153S–1161S.
5. Jolliffe N and Archer M. Statistical associations between international coronary heart disease death rates and certain environmental factors. *Journal of Chronic Diseases* 1959;9:636–652.
6. Scrimgeour EM, McCall MG, Smith DE, and Masarei JR. Levels of serum cholesterol, triglyceride, HDL-cholesterol, apoproteins A-I and B, and plasma glucose, and prevalence of diastolic hypertension and cigarette smoking in Papua New Guinea highlanders. *Pathology* 1989;21:46–50.
7. Campbell TC, Parpia B, and Chen J. Diet, lifestyle, and the etiology of coronary artery disease: The Cornell China study. *American Journal of Cardiology* 1998;82:18T–21T.
8. Ornish D, Scherwitz LW, Billings JH, Gould L, et al. Intensive lifestyle changes for reversal of coronary heart disease. *JAMA: The Journal of the American Medical Association* 1998;280:2001–2007.
9. Himsworth H. Diet and the incidence of diabetes mellitus. *Clinical Science* 1935;2:117–148.
10. Barnard RJ, Lattimore L, Holly RG, Cherny S, and Pritikin N. Response of non-insulin-dependent diabetic patients to an intensive program of diet and exercise. *Diabetes Care* 1982;5:370–374.
11. Fraser GE. Vegetarian diets: What do we know of their effects on common chronic diseases? *American Journal of Clinical Nutrition* 2009;89:1607S–1612S.
12. Newby PK, Tucker KL, and Wolk A. Risk of overweight and obesity among semivegetarian, lactovegetarian, and vegan women. *American Journal of Clinical Nutrition* 2005;81:1267–1274.
13. Dwyer JT. Health aspects of vegetarian diets. *American Journal of Clinical Nutrition* 1988;48:712–738.
14. Vergnaud AC, Norat T, Romaguera D, Mouw T, et al. Meat consumption and prospective weight change in participants of the EPIC-PANACEA study. *American Journal of Clinical Nutrition* 2010;92:398–407.
15. Campbell TM 2nd and Campbell TC. The breadth of evidence favoring a whole foods, plant-based diet: Part I: Metabolic diseases and diseases of aging. *Primary Care Reports* 2012;18:13–23.
16. Barnard ND, Cohen J, Jenkins DJA, Turner-McGrievy G, et al. A low-fat vegan diet and a conventional diabetes diet in the treatment of type 2 diabetes: A randomized, controlled, 74-wk clinical trial. *American Journal of Clinical Nutrition* 2009;89:1588S–1596S.

17. Ornish D, Weidner G, Fair WR, Marlin R, et al. Intensive lifestyle changes may affect the progression of prostate cancer. *Journal of Urology* 2005;174:1065–1069.

18. Ornish D, Magbanua MJM, Weidner G, Weinberg V, et al. Changes in prostate gene expression in men undergoing an intensive nutrition and lifestyle intervention. *Proceedings of the National Academy of Sciences of the United States of America* 2008;105:8369–8374.

19. Ornish D, Lin J, Chan JM, Epel E, et al. Effect of comprehensive lifestyle changes on telomerase activity and telomere length in men with biopsy-proven low-risk prostate cancer: 5-year follow-up of a descriptive pilot study. *Lancet Oncology* 2013;14:1112–1120.

20. Brown K, DeCoffe D, Molcan E, and Gibson DL. Diet-induced dysbiosis of the intestinal microbiota and the effects on immunity and disease. *Nutrients* 2012;4:1095–1119.

21. Zhang C, Zhang M, Wang S, Han R, et al. Interactions between gut microbiota, host genetics and diet relevant to development of metabolic syndromes in mice. *ISME Journal* 2010;4:232–241.

22. De Filippo C, Cavalieri D, Di Paola M, Ramazzotti M, et al. Impact of diet in shaping gut microbiota revealed by a comparative study in children from Europe and rural Africa. *Proceedings of the National Academy of Sciences of the United States of America* 2010;107:14691–14696.

23. Turnbaugh PJ, Ridaura VK, Faith JJ, Rey FE, et al. The effect of diet on the human gut microbiome: A metagenomic analysis in humanized gnotobiotic mice. *Science Translational Medicine* 2009;1:6ra14.

24. Koeth RA, Wang Z, Levison BS, Buffa JA, et al. Intestinal microbiota metabolism of L-carnitine, a nutrient in red meat, promotes atherosclerosis. *Nature Medicine* 2013;19:576–585.

CHAPTER 2

1. Varki N, Anderson D, Herndon JG, Gregg, CJ, et al. Heart disease is common in humans and chimpanzees, but is caused by different pathological processes. *Evolutionary Applications* 2009;2:101–112.

2. Popovich DG and Dierenfeld ES. Gorilla nutrition. In: Ogden J and Wharton D, eds. *Management of gorillas in captivity: Husbandry manual, Gorilla Species Survival Plan.* Atlanta: Gorilla Species Survival Plan and Atlanta/Fulton County Zoo, Inc., 1997.

3. Less EH. "Adiposity in zoo gorillas (*Gorilla gorilla gorilla*): The effects of diet and behavior" (PhD dissertation, Case Western Reserve University, 2012), https://etd.ohiolink.edu/rws_etd/document/get/case1322582620/inline.

4. Popovich DG, Jenkins DJA, Kendall CWC, Dierenfeld ES, et al. The western lowland gorilla diet has implications for the health of humans and other hominoids. *Journal of Nutrition* 1997;127:2000–2005.

5. Schmidt DA, Ellersieck MR, Cranfield MR, and Karesh WB. Cholesterol values in free-ranging gorillas (*Gorilla gorilla gorilla* and *Gorilla beringei*) and Bornean orangutans (*Pongo pygmaeus*). *Journal of Zoo and Wildlife Medicine* 2006;37:292–300.

6. Eaton SB, Cordain L, and Lindeberg S. Evolutionary health promotion: A consideration of common counterarguments. *Preventive Medicine* 2002;34:119–123.

7. Caspari R and Lee SH. Older age becomes common late in human evolution. *Proceedings of the National Academy of Sciences of the United States of America* 2004;101:10895–10900.

8. Trinkaus E. Late Pleistocene adult mortality patterns and modern human establishment. *Proceedings of the National Academy of Sciences of the United States of America* 2011;108:1267–1271.

9. Cordain L, Miller JB, Eaton SB, Mann N, et al. Plant-animal subsistence ratios and macronutrient energy estimations in worldwide hunter-gatherer diets. *American Journal of Clinical Nutrition* 2000;71:682–692.

10. Murdock GP. Ethnographic Atlas: A summary. *Ethnology* 1967;6:109–236.

11. Cordain L. *The Paleo diet: Lose weight and get healthy by eating the foods you were designed to eat* (rev. ed.). Hoboken, NJ: Wiley, 2011.

12. National Cancer Institute. Table 1A: Mean intake of energy and percentage contribution of various foods among US population, by age, NHANES 2005–06. October 18, 2013. http://appliedresearch.cancer.gov/diet/foodsources/energy/table1a.html. http://appliedresearch.cancer.gov/diet/foodsources/energy/table1a.html.

13. Frassetto LA, Schloetter M, Mietus-Synder M, Morris RC Jr., and Sebastian A. Metabolic and physiologic improvements from consuming a Paleolithic, hunter-gatherer type diet. *European Journal of Clinical Nutrition* 2009;63:947–955.

14. Jönsson T, Granfeldt Y, Ahrén B, Branell UC, et al. Beneficial effects of a Paleolithic diet on cardiovascular risk factors in type 2 diabetes: A randomized cross-over pilot study. *Cardiovascular Diabetology* 2009;8:35.

15. Lindeberg S, Jönsson T, Granfeldt Y, Borgstrand E, et al. A Palaeolithic diet improves glucose tolerance more than a Mediterranean-like diet in individuals with ischaemic heart disease. *Diabetologia* 2007;50:1795–1807.

16. Osterdahl M, Kocturk T, Koochek A, and Wandell PE. Effects of a short-term intervention with a Paleolithic diet in healthy volunteers. *European Journal of Clinical Nutrition* 2008;62:682–685.

17. Milton K. Hunter-gatherer diets—A different perspective. *American Journal of Clinical Nutrition* 2000;71:665–667.

18. Eaton SB and Konner M. Paleolithic nutrition: A consideration of its nature and current implications. *New England Journal of Medicine* 1985;312:283–289.

19. Richards MP. A brief review of the archaeological evidence for Palaeolithic and Neolithic subsistence. *European Journal of Clinical Nutrition* 2002;56:1270–1278.

20. Warinner C, Robles-Garcia N, and Tuross N. *The isotopic diversity of the Middle American Dietome: Implications for Paleodiet reconstruction and the origins of maize agriculture.* Poster presentation at the UK Archaeological Science Biennial Conference, September 8–10, 2009, Nottingham, England.

21. Warinner C. "Life and death at Teposcolula Yucundaa: Mortuary, archaeogenetic, and isotopic investigations of the early colonial period in Mexico" (PhD dissertation, Harvard University, 2010), http://christinawarinner.com/wp-content/uploads/2012/02/Warinner_Dissertation_June252010.pdf.

22. Warinner C. "Debunking the Paleo Diet." Filmed 2012. TEDxOU video, 22:18. Posted February 12, 2013. https://www.youtube.com/watch?v=BMOjVYgYaG8.

23. Henry AG, Brooks AS, and Piperno DR. Microfossils in calculus demonstrate consumption of plants and cooked foods in Neanderthal diets (Shanidar III, Iraq; Spy I and II, Belgium). *Proceedings of the National Academy of Sciences of the United States of America* 2011;108:486–491.

24. Liu L, Bestel S, Shi J, Song Y, and Chen X. Paleolithic human exploitation of plant foods during the last glacial maximum in North China. *Proceedings of the National Academy of Sciences of the United States of America* 2013;110:5380–5385.

25. Mercader J. Mozambican grass seed consumption during the Middle Stone Age. *Science* 2009;326:1680–1683.

26. Sponheimer M, Alemseged Z, Cerling TE, Grine FE, et al. Isotopic evidence of early hominin diets. *Proceedings of the National Academy of Sciences of the United States of America* 2013;110:10513–10518.

27. Carroll KK. Experimental evidence of dietary factors and hormone-dependent cancers. *Cancer Research* 1975;35:3374–3383.

28. Cerling TE, Manthi FK, Mbua EN, et al. Stable isotope-based diet reconstructions of Turkana Basin hominins. *Proceedings of the National Academy of Sciences of the United States of America* 2013;110:10501–10506.

29. Himsworth H. Diet and the incidence of diabetes mellitus. *Clinical Science* 1935;2:117–148.

30. Berkow SE and Barnard N. Vegetarian diets and weight status. *Nutrition Reviews* 2006;64:175–188.

31. Vergnaud A-C, Norat T, Romaguera D, Mouw T, et al. Meat consumption and prospective weight change in participants of the EPIC-PANACEA study. *American Journal of Clinical Nutrition* 2010;92:398–407.

32. Ornish D, Scherwitz LW, Billings JH, Gould L, et al. Intensive lifestyle changes for reversal of coronary heart disease. *JAMA: The Journal of the American Medical Association* 1998;280:2001–2007.

33. Esselstyn CB Jr., Ellis SG, Medendorp SV, and Crowe TD. A strategy to arrest and reverse coronary artery disease: A 5-year longitudinal study of a single physician's practice. *Journal of Family Practice* 1995;41:560–568.

34. Barnard ND, Cohen J, Jenkins DJA, Turner-McGrievy G, et al. A low-fat vegan diet improves glycemic control and cardiovascular risk factors in a randomized clinical trial in individuals with type 2 diabetes. *Diabetes Care* 2006;29:1777–1783.

35. Barnard RJ, Massey MR, Cherny S, O'Brien LT, and Pritikin N. Long-term use of a high-complex-carbohydrate, high-fiber, low-fat diet and exercise in the treatment of NIDDM patients. *Diabetes Care* 1983;6:268–273.

36. Ornish D, Magbanua MJM, Weidner G, Weinberg V, et al. Changes in prostate gene expression in men undergoing an intensive nutrition and lifestyle intervention. *Proceedings of the National Academy of Sciences of the United States of America* 2008;105:8369–8374.

37. Ornish D, Weidner G, Fair WR, Marlin R, et al. Intensive lifestyle changes may affect the progression of prostate cancer. *Journal of Urology* 2005;174:1065–1069.

38. Jenkins DJA, Kendall CWC, Augustin LSA, Mitchell S, et al. Effect of legumes as part of a low glycemic index diet on glycemic control and cardiovascular risk factors in type 2 diabetes mellitus: A randomized controlled trial. *Archives of Internal Medicine* 2012;172:1653–1660.

39. Cho SS, Qi L, Fahey GC Jr., and Klurfeld DM. Consumption of cereal fiber, mixtures of whole grains and bran, and whole grains and risk reduction in type 2 diabetes, obesity, and cardiovascular disease. *American Journal of Clinical Nutrition* 2013;98:594–619.

40. Slavin JL, Jacobs D, Marquart L, and Wiemer K. The role of whole grains in disease prevention. *Journal of the American Dietetic Association* 2001;101:780–785.

41. Anderson JW and Ward K. High-carbohydrate, high-fiber diets for insulin-treated men with diabetes mellitus. *American Journal of Clinical Nutrition* 1979;32:2312–2321.

42. Youngman LD and Campbell TC. Inhibition of aflatoxin B1-induced gamma-glutamyltranspeptidase positive (GGT+) hepatic preneoplastic foci and tumors by low protein diets: Evidence that altered GGT+ foci indicate neoplastic potential. *Carcinogenesis* 1992;13:1607–1613.

43. Addis T. *Glomerular nephritis: Diagnosis and treatment.* New York: Macmillan, 1948.

44. Fouque D and Aparicio M. Eleven reasons to control the protein intake of patients with chronic kidney disease. *Nature Clinical Practice: Nephrology* 2007;3:383–392.

45. Hostetter TH, Olson JL, Rennke HG, Venkatachalam MA, and Brenner BM. Hyperfiltration in remnant nephrons: A potentially adverse response to renal ablation. *Journal of the American Society of Nephrology* 2001;12:1315–1325.

46. Kritchevsky D and Klurfeld DM. Gallstone formation in hamsters: Effect of varying animal and vegetable protein levels. *American Journal of Clinical Nutrition* 1983;37:802–804.

47. Foo SY, Heller ER, Wykrzykowska J, Sullivan CJ, et al. Vascular effects of a low-carbohydrate high-protein diet. *Proceedings of the National Academy of Sciences of the United States of America* 2009;106:15418–15423.

48. Koeth RA, Wang Z, Levison BS, Buffa JA, et al. Intestinal microbiota metabolism of L-carnitine, a nutrient in red meat, promotes atherosclerosis. *Nature Medicine* 2013;19:576–585.

49. Aune D, Ursin G, and Veierod MB. Meat consumption and the risk of type 2 diabetes: A systematic review and meta-analysis of cohort studies. *Diabetologia* 2009;52:2277–2287.

50. Lagiou P, Sandin S, Weiderpass E, Lagiou A, et al. Low carbohydrate–high protein diet and mortality in a cohort of Swedish women. *Journal of Internal Medicine* 2007;261:366–374.

51. Trichopoulou A, Psaltopoulou T, Orfanos P, Hsieh CC, and Trichopoulos D. Low-carbohydrate-high-protein diet and long-term survival in a general population cohort. *European Journal of Clinical Nutrition* 2007;61:575–581.

52. Agatston A. *The South Beach Diet: The delicious, doctor-designed, foolproof plan for fast and healthy weight loss.* Emmaus, PA: Rodale, 2003.

53. Ornish D, Brown SE, Billings JH, Scherwitz LW, et al. Can lifestyle changes reverse coronary heart disease? [see comment]. *Lancet* 1990;336:129–133.

54. Esselstyn CB Jr. Updating a 12-year experience with arrest and reversal therapy for coronary heart disease (an overdue requiem for palliative cardiology). *American Journal of Cardiology* 1999;84:339–341, A8.

55. Hite AH, Berkowitz VG, and Berkowitz K. Low-carbohydrate diet review: Shifting the paradigm. *Nutrition in Clinical Practice* 2011;26:300–308.

56. Smith SR. A look at the low-carbohydrate diet. *New England Journal of Medicine* 2009;361:2286–2288.

57. Merino J, Kones R, Ferré R, Plana N, et al. Negative effect of a low-carbohydrate, high-protein, high-fat diet on small peripheral artery reactivity in patients with increased cardiovascular risk. *British Journal of Nutrition* 2013;109:1241–1247.

58. de Koning L, Fung TT, Liao X, Chiuve SE, et al. Low-carbohydrate diet scores and risk of type 2 diabetes in men. *American Journal of Clinical Nutrition* 2011;93:844–850.

59. Sjögren P, Becker W, Warensjö E, Olsson E, et al. Mediterranean and carbohydrate-restricted diets and mortality among elderly men: A cohort study in Sweden. *American Journal of Clinical Nutrition* 2010;92:967–974.

60. Fung TT, van Dam RM, Hankinson SE, Stampfer M, et al. Low-carbohydrate diets and all-cause and cause-specific mortality: Two cohort studies. *Annals of Internal Medicine* 2010;153:289–298.

CHAPTER 3

1. Rothman JM, Raubenheimer D, and Chapman CA. Nutritional geometry: Gorillas prioritize non-protein energy while consuming surplus protein. *Biology Letters* 2011;7:847–849.

2. Tonstad S, Butler T, Yan R, and Fraser GE. Type of vegetarian diet, body weight, and prevalence of type 2 diabetes. *Diabetes Care* 2009;32:791–796.

3. Davey GK, Spencer EA, Appleby PN, Allen NE, et al. EPIC–Oxford: Lifestyle characteristics and nutrient intakes in a cohort of 33,883 meat-eaters and 31,546 non meat-eaters in the UK. *Public Health Nutrition* 2003;6:259–269.

4. Fraser GE. Vegetarian diets: What do we know of their effects on common chronic diseases? *American Journal of Clinical Nutrition* 2009;89:1607S–1612S.

5. Bradbury KE, Crowe FL, Appleby PN, Schmidt JA, et al. Serum concentrations of cholesterol, apolipoprotein A-I and apolipoprotein B in a total of 1694 meat-eaters, fish-eaters, vegetarians and vegans. *European Journal of Clinical Nutrition* 2014;68:178–183.

CHAPTER 4

1. Campbell TC and Junshi C. Diet and chronic degenerative diseases: Perspectives from China. *American Journal of Clinical Nutrition* 1994;59:1153S–1161S.

2. Campbell TC, Parpia B, and Chen J. Diet, lifestyle, and the etiology of coronary artery disease: The Cornell China study. *American Journal of Cardiology* 1998;82:18T–21T.

3. de Lorgeril M, Renaud S, Salen P, Monjaud I, et al. Mediterranean alpha-linolenic acid-rich diet in secondary prevention of coronary heart disease. *Lancet* 1994;343:1454–1459.

4. de Lorgeril M, Salen P, Martin J-L, Monjaud I, et al. Mediterranean diet, traditional risk factors, and the rate of cardiovascular complications after myocardial infarction: Final report of the Lyon Diet Heart Study. *Circulation* 1999;99:779–785.

5. Singh RB, Rastogi SS, Verma R, Laxmi B, et al. Randomised controlled trial of cardioprotective diet in patients with recent acute myocardial infarction: Results of one year follow up. *BMJ* 1992;304:1015–1019.

6. Esselstyn CB Jr., Ellis SG, Medendorp SV, and Crowe TD. A strategy to arrest and reverse coronary artery disease: A 5-year longitudinal study of a single physician's practice. *Journal of Family Practice* 1995;41:560–568.

7. Ornish D, Scherwitz LW, Billings JH, Gould L, et al. Intensive lifestyle changes for reversal of coronary heart disease. *JAMA: The Journal of the American Medical Association* 1998;280:2001–2007.

8. Esselstyn CB Jr. Resolving the coronary artery disease epidemic through plant-based nutrition. *Preventive Cardiology* 2001;4:171–177.

9. Pierce JP, Natarajan L, Caan BJ, Parker BA, et al. Influence of a diet very high in vegetables, fruit, and fiber and low in fat on prognosis following treatment for breast cancer: The Women's Healthy Eating and Living (WHEL) randomized trial. *JAMA: The Journal of the American Medical Association* 2007;298:289–298.

10. Smith-Warner SA, Spiegelman D, Yaun S-S, Adami H-O, et al. Intake of fruits and vegetables and risk of breast cancer: A pooled analysis of cohort studies. *JAMA: The Journal of the American Medical Association* 2001;285:769–776.

11. van Gils CH, Peeters PHM, Bueno-de-Mesquita HB, Boshuizen HC, et al. Consumption of vegetables and fruits and risk of breast cancer. *JAMA: The Journal of the American Medical Association* 2005;293:183–193.

12. Prentice RL, Thomson CA, Caan B, Hubbell FA, et al. Low-fat dietary pattern and cancer incidence in the Women's Health Initiative Dietary Modification Randomized Controlled Trial. *Journal of the National Cancer Institute* 2007;99:1534–1543.

13. Prentice RL, Caan B, Chlebowski RT, Patterson R, et al. Low-fat dietary pattern and risk of invasive breast cancer: The Women's Health Initiative Randomized Controlled Dietary Modification Trial. *JAMA: The Journal of the American Medical Association* 2006;295:629–642.

14. Beresford SAA, Johnson KC, Ritenbaugh C, Lasser NL, et al. Low-fat dietary pattern and risk of colorectal cancer: The Women's Health Initiative Randomized Controlled Dietary Modification Trial. *JAMA: The Journal of the American Medical Association* 2006;295:643–654.

15. Avena NM, Rada P, and Hoebel BG. Sugar and fat bingeing have notable differences in addictive-like behavior. *Journal of Nutrition* 2009;139:623–628.

16. Kelley AE, Bakshi VP, Haber SN, Steininger TL, et al. Opioid modulation of taste hedonics within the ventral striatum. *Physiology and Behavior* 2002;76:365–377.

17. Lenoir M, Serre F, Cantin L, and Ahmed SH. Intense sweetness surpasses cocaine reward. *PloS One* 2007;2:e698.

18. Berner LA, Avena NM, and Hoebel BG. Bingeing, self-restriction, and increased body weight in rats with limited access to a sweet-fat diet. *Obesity* 2008;16:1998–2002.

CHAPTER 5

1. Applied Research Program, National Cancer Institute. Usual intake of added sugars, 2001–2004. April 2, 2014. http://riskfactor.cancer.gov/diet/usualintakes/pop/added_sugars.html.

2. Applied Research Program, National Cancer Institute. Added sugars, 2001–2004. October 18, 2013. http://riskfactor.cancer.gov/diet/usualintakes/addedsugars.html.

3. Applied Research Program, National Cancer Institute. Usual intake of dark-green vegetables, 2001–2004. April 2, 2014. http://riskfactor.cancer.gov/diet/usualintakes/pop/veg_drkgreen.html.

4. Johnson RK, Appel LJ, Brands M, Howard BV, et al. Dietary sugars intake and cardiovascular health: A scientific statement from the American Heart Association. *Circulation* 2009;120:1011–1020.

5. Guthrie JF and Morton JF. Food sources of added sweeteners in the diets of Americans. *Journal of the American Dietetic Association* 2000;100:43–51.

6. Avena NM, Rada P, and Hoebel BG. Sugar and fat bingeing have notable differences in addictive-like behavior. *Journal of Nutrition* 2009;139:623–628.

7. Kranz S, Smiciklas-Wright H, Siega-Riz AM, and Mitchell D. Adverse effect of high added sugar consumption on dietary intake in American preschoolers. *Journal of Pediatrics* 2005;146:105–111.

8. Vartanian LR, Schwartz MB, and Brownell KD. Effects of soft drink consumption on nutrition and health: A systematic review and meta-analysis. *American Journal of Public Health* 2007;97:667–675.

9. Malik VS and Hu FB. Sweeteners and risk of obesity and type 2 diabetes: The role of sugar-sweetened beverages. *Current Diabetes Reports* 2012;12:195–203.

10. Curhan GC and Forman JP. Sugar-sweetened beverages and chronic disease. *Kidney International* 2010;77:569–570.

11. Gaby AR. Nutritional approaches to prevention and treatment of gallstones. *Alternative Medicine Review* 2009;14:258–267.

12. Zero DT. Sugars—The arch criminal? *Caries Research* 2004;38:277–285.

13. Yang Q. Gain weight by "going diet?" Artificial sweeteners and the neurobiology of sugar cravings: Neuroscience 2010. *Yale Journal of Biology and Medicine* 2010;83:101–108.

14. Messina MJ and Wood CE. Soy isoflavones, estrogen therapy, and breast cancer risk: Analysis and commentary. *Nutrition Journal* 2008;7:17.

15. de Cremoux P, This P, Leclercq G, and Jacquot Y. Controversies concerning the use of phytoestrogens in menopause management: Bioavailability and metabolism. *Maturitas* 2010;65:334–339.

16. Wu AH, Pike MC, and Stram DO. Meta-analysis: Dietary fat intake, serum estrogen levels, and the risk of breast cancer. *Journal of the National Cancer Institute* 1999;91:529–534.

17. Krebs EE, Ensrud KE, MacDonald R, and Wilt TJ. Phytoestrogens for treatment of menopausal symptoms: A systematic review. *Obstetrics and Gynecology* 2004;104:824–836.

18. Tempfer CB, Froese G, Heinze G, Bentz EK, et al. Side effects of phytoestrogens: A meta-analysis of randomized trials. *American Journal of Medicine* 2009;122:939–946.e9.

19. Hamilton-Reeves JM, Vazquez G, Duval SJ, Phipps WR, et al. Clinical studies show no effects of soy protein or isoflavones on reproductive hormones in men: Results of a meta-analysis. *Fertility and Sterility* 2010;94:997–1007.

20. Cederroth CR, Auger J, Zimmermann C, Eustache F, and Nef S. Soy, phyto-oestrogens and male reproductive function: A review. *International Journal of Andrology* 2010;33:304–316.

CHAPTER 6

1. Harvard School of Public Health. The Nutrition Source: What should I eat? Fats and cholesterol. n.d. www.hsph.harvard.edu/nutritionsource/what-should-you-eat/fats-and-cholesterol/index.html.

2. Harvard School of Public Health. The Nutrition Source: What should I eat? Healthy Eating Plate and Healthy Eating Pyramid. n.d. www.hsph.harvard.edu/nutritionsource/what-should-you-eat/pyramid/index.html.

3. Chowdhury R, Warnakula S, Kunutsor S, Crowe F, et al. Association of dietary, circulating, and supplement fatty acids with coronary risk: A systematic review and meta-analysis. *Annals of Internal Medicine* 2014;160:398–406.

4. Martin A. The colonel is phasing out trans fat from the menu. *New York Times,* October 31, 2006.

5. Beating Edge Team. Health Hub: Heart-healthy cooking: Oils 101. Cleveland Clinic Health, May 31, 2012. http://cchealth.clevelandclinic.org/heart-health/heart-healthy-cooking-oils-101.

6. Carroll KK, Gammal EB, and Plunkett ER. Dietary fat and mammary cancer. *Canadian Medical Association Journal* 1968;98:590–594.

7. National Research Council. *Diet, nutrition, and cancer.* Washington, DC: National Academies Press, 1982.

8. Jolliffe N and Archer M. Statistical associations between international coronary heart disease death rates and certain environmental factors. *Journal of Chronic Diseases* 1959;9:636–652.

9. Keys A. Diet and the epidemiology of coronary heart disease. *Journal of the American Medical Association* 1957;164:1912–1919.

10. Bang HO, Dyerberg J, and Hjoorne N. The composition of food consumed by Greenland Eskimos. *Acta Medica Scandinavica* 1976;200:69–73.

11. Bjerregaard P, Young TK, and Hegele RA. Low incidence of cardiovascular disease among the Inuit—What is the evidence? *Atherosclerosis* 2003;166:351–357.

12. Bang HO, Dyerberg J, and Nielsen AB. Plasma lipid and lipoprotein pattern in Greenlandic west-coast Eskimos. *Lancet* 1971;1:1143–1145.

13. Bang HO, Dyerberg J, and Sinclair HM. The composition of the Eskimo food in north western Greenland. *American Journal of Clinical Nutrition* 1980;33:2657–2661.

14. Keys A, Mienotti A, Karvonen MJ, Aravanis C, et al. The diet and 15-year death rate in the Seven Countries Study. *American Journal of Epidemiology* 1986;124:903–915.

15. Kromhout D, Bosschieter EB, and de Lezenne Coulander C. The inverse relation between fish consumption and 20-year mortality from coronary heart disease. *New England Journal of Medicine* 1985;312:1205–1209.

16. He K, Song Y, Daviglus ML, Liu K, et al. Accumulated evidence on fish consumption and coronary heart disease mortality: A meta-analysis of cohort studies. *Circulation* 2004;109:2705–2711.

17. Breslow JL. n-3 Fatty acids and cardiovascular disease. *American Journal of Clinical Nutrition* 2006;83:1477S–1482S.

18. Mozaffarian D and Wu JH. Omega-3 fatty acids and cardiovascular disease: Effects on risk factors, molecular pathways, and clinical events. *Journal of the American College of Cardiology* 2011;58:2047–2067.

19. Sofi F, Abbate R, Gensini GF, and Casini A. Accruing evidence on benefits of adherence to the Mediterranean diet on health: An updated systematic review and meta-analysis. *American Journal of Clinical Nutrition* 2010;92:1189–1196.

20. Sofi F, Cesari F, Abbate R, Gensini GF, and Casini A. Adherence to Mediterranean diet and health status: Meta-analysis. *BMJ* 2008;337:a1344.

21. Oomen CM, Feskens EJ, Räsänen L, Fidanza F, et al. Fish consumption and coronary heart disease mortality in Finland, Italy, and the Netherlands. *American Journal of Epidemiology* 2000;151:999–1006.

22. Virtanen JK, Mozaffarian D, Chiuve SE, and Rimm EB. Fish consumption and risk of major chronic disease in men. *American Journal of Clinical Nutrition* 2008;88:1618–1625.

23. Estruch R, Ros E, Salas-Salvadó J, Covas M-I, et al. Primary prevention of cardiovascular disease with a Mediterranean diet. *New England Journal of Medicine* 2013;368:1279–1290.

24. Marchioli R, Barzi F, Bomba E, Chieffo C, et al. Early protection against sudden death by n-3 polyunsaturated fatty acids after myocardial infarction: Time-course analysis of the results of the Gruppo Italiano per lo Studio della Sopravvivenza nell'Infarto Miocardico (GISSI)-Prevenzione. *Circulation* 2002;105:1897–1903.

25. Burr ML. Secondary prevention of CHD in UK men: The Diet and Reinfarction Trial and its sequel. *Proceedings of the Nutrition Society* 2007;66:9–15.

26. Yokoyama M, Origasa H, Matsuzaki M, Matsuzawa Y, et al. Effects of eicosapentaenoic acid on major coronary events in hypercholesterolaemic patients (JELIS): A randomised open-label, blinded endpoint analysis. *Lancet* 2007;369:1090–1098.

27. Rizos EC, Ntzani EE, Bika E, Kostapanos MS, and Elisaf MS. Association between omega-3 fatty acid supplementation and risk of major cardiovascular disease events: A systematic review and meta-analysis. *JAMA: The Journal of the American Medical Association* 2012;308:1024–1033.

28. Hooper L, Thompson RL, Harrison RA, Summerbell CD, et al. Risks and benefits of omega 3 fats for mortality, cardiovascular disease, and cancer: Systematic review. *BMJ* 2006;332:752–760.

29. Artaud-Wild SM, Connor SL, Sexton G, and Connor WE. Differences in coronary mortality can be explained by differences in cholesterol and saturated fat intakes in 40 countries but not in France and Finland: A paradox. *Circulation* 1993;88:2771–2779.

30. Campbell TC, Parpia B, and Chen J. Diet, lifestyle, and the etiology of coronary artery disease: The Cornell China study. *American Journal of Cardiology* 1998;82:18T–21T.

31. Randi G, Pelucchi C, Gallus S, Parpinel M, et al. Lipid, protein and carbohydrate intake in relation to body mass index: An Italian study. *Public Health Nutrition* 2007;10:306–310.

32. Trichopoulou A, Gnardellis C, Benetou V, Lagiou P, et al. Lipid, protein and carbohydrate intake in relation to body mass index. *European Journal of Clinical Nutrition* 2002;56:37–43.

33. Gosmanov AR, Smiley DD, Robalino G, Siquiera J, et al. Effects of oral and intravenous fat load on blood pressure, endothelial function, sympathetic activity, and oxidative stress in obese healthy subjects. *American Journal of Physiology: Endocrinology and Metabolism* 2010;299:E953–E958.

34. Gokce N, Keaney JF Jr., Hunter LM, Watkins MT, et al. Risk stratification for postoperative cardiovascular events via noninvasive assessment of endothelial function: A prospective study. *Circulation* 2002;105:1567–1572.

35. Neunteufl T, Heher S, Katzenschlager R, Wölfl G, et al. Late prognostic value of flow-mediated dilation in the brachial artery of patients with chest pain. *American Journal of Cardiology* 2000;86:207–210.

36. Amir O, Jaffe R, Shiran A, Flugelman MY, et al. Brachial reactivity and extent of coronary artery disease in patients with first ST-elevation acute myocardial infarction. *American Journal of Cardiology* 2006;98:754–757.

37. Landmesser U, Hornig B, and Drexler H. Endothelial function: A critical determinant in atherosclerosis? *Circulation* 2004;109:II27–II33.

38. Cuevas AM, Guasch V, Castillo O, Irribarra V, et al. A high-fat diet induces and red wine counteracts endothelial dysfunction in human volunteers. *Lipids* 2000;35:143–148.

39. Ong PJ, Dean TS, Hayward CS, Della Monica PL, et al. Effect of fat and carbohydrate consumption on endothelial function. *Lancet* 1999;354:2134.

40. Vogel RA, Corretti MC, and Plotnick GD. Effect of a single high-fat meal on endothelial function in healthy subjects. *American Journal of Cardiology* 1997;79:350–354.

41. Marchesi S, Lupattelli G, Schillaci G, Pirro M, et al. Impaired flow-mediated vasoactivity during post-prandial phase in young healthy men. *Atherosclerosis* 2000;153:397–402.

42. Bae J-H, Schwemmer M, Lee I-K, Lee H-J, et al. Postprandial hypertriglyceridemia-induced endothelial dysfunction in healthy subjects is independent of lipid oxidation. *International Journal of Cardiology* 2003;87:259–267.

43. Blankenhorn DH, Johnson RL, Mack WJ, el Zein HA, and Vailas LI. The influence of diet on the appearance of new lesions in human coronary arteries. *JAMA: The Journal of the American Medical Association* 1990;263:1646–1652.

44. Ornish D, Brown SE, Billings JH, Scherwitz LW, et al. Can lifestyle changes reverse coronary heart disease? The Lifestyle Heart Trial. *Lancet* 1990;336:129–133.

45. Ornish D, Scherwitz LW, Billings JH, Gould L, et al. Intensive lifestyle changes for reversal of coronary heart disease. *JAMA: The Journal of the American Medical Association* 1998;280:2001–2007.

46. Esselstyn CB Jr. Updating a 12-year experience with arrest and reversal therapy for coronary heart disease (an overdue requiem for palliative cardiology). *American Journal of Cardiology* 1999;84:339–341.

47. Esselstyn CB Jr., Ellis SG, Medendorp SV, and Crowe TD. A strategy to arrest and reverse coronary artery disease: A 5-year longitudinal study of a single physician's practice. *Journal of Family Practice* 1995;41:560–568.

CHAPTER 7

1. Kris-Etherton PM, Harris WS, and Appel LJ. Fish consumption, fish oil, omega-3 fatty acids, and cardiovascular disease. *Circulation* 2002;106:2747–2757.

2. Daviglus ML, Stamler J, Orencia AJ, Dyer AR, et al. Fish consumption and the 30-year risk of fatal myocardial infarction. *New England Journal of Medicine* 1997;336:1046–1053.

3. He K, Song Y, Daviglus ML, Liu K, et al. Accumulated evidence on fish consumption and coronary heart disease mortality: A meta-analysis of cohort studies. *Circulation* 2004;109:2705–2711.

4. Heine-Bröring RC, Brouwer IA, Proençca RV, van Rooij FJA, et al. Intake of fish and marine n-3 fatty acids in relation to coronary calcification: The Rotterdam Study. *American Journal of Clinical Nutrition* 2010;91:1317–1323.

5. Hu FB, Bronner L, Willett WC, Stampfer MJ, et al. Fish and omega-3 fatty acid intake and risk of coronary heart disease in women. *JAMA: The Journal of the American Medical Association* 2002;287:1815–1821.

6. Kromhout D, Bosschieter EB, and de Lezenne Coulander C. The inverse relation between fish consumption and 20-year mortality from coronary heart disease. *New England Journal of Medicine* 1985;312:1205–1209.

7. Kromhout D, Feskens EJ, and Bowles CH. The protective effect of a small amount of fish on coronary heart disease mortality in an elderly population. *International Journal of Epidemiology* 1995;24:340–345.

8. Shekelle R, Missell L, Paul O, Shryock A, and Stamler J. Fish consumption and mortality from coronary heart disease. *New England Journal of Medicine* 1985;313:820–824.

9. Zhang J, Sasaki S, Amano K, and Kesteloot H. Fish consumption and mortality from all causes, ischemic heart disease, and stroke: An ecological study. *Preventive Medicine* 1999;28:520–529.

10. Virtanen JK, Mozaffarian D, Chiuve SE, and Rimm EB. Fish consumption and risk of major chronic disease in men. *American Journal of Clinical Nutrition* 2008;88:1618–1625.

11. Mozaffarian D, Lemaitre RN, Kuller LH, Burke GL, et al. Cardiac benefits of fish consumption may depend on the type of fish meal consumed: The Cardiovascular Health Study. *Circulation* 2003;107:1372–1377.

12. Strom M, Halldorsson TI, Mortensen EL, Torp-Pedersen C, and Olsen SF. Fish, n-3 fatty acids, and cardiovascular diseases in women of reproductive age: A prospective study in a large national cohort. *Hypertension* 2012;59:36–43.

13. Oomen CM, Feskens EJ, Räsänen L, Fidanza F, et al. Fish consumption and coronary heart disease mortality in Finland, Italy, and the Netherlands. *American Journal of Epidemiology* 2000;151:999–1006.

14. Mizushima S, Moriguchi EH, Ishikawa P, Hekman P, et al. Fish intake and cardiovascular risk among middle-aged Japanese in Japan and Brazil. *Journal of Cardiovascular Risk* 1997;4:191–199.

15. Rizos EC, Ntzani EE, Bika E, Kostapanos MS, and Elisaf MS. Association between omega-3 fatty acid supplementation and risk of major cardiovascular disease events: A systematic review and meta-analysis. *JAMA: The Journal of the American Medical Association* 2012;308:1024–1033.

16. Kaushik M, Mozaffarian D, Spiegelman D, Manson JE, et al. Long-chain omega-3 fatty acids, fish intake, and the risk of type 2 diabetes mellitus. *American Journal of Clinical Nutrition* 2009;90:613–620.

17. Miles EA and Calder PC. Influence of marine n-3 polyunsaturated fatty acids on immune function and a systematic review of their effects on clinical outcomes in rheumatoid arthritis. *British Journal of Nutrition* 2012;107 Suppl 2:S171–S184.

18. Rangel-Huerta OD, Aguilera CM, Mesa MD, and Gil A. Omega-3 long-chain polyunsaturated fatty acids supplementation on inflammatory biomarkers: A systematic review of randomised clinical trials. *British Journal of Nutrition* 2012;107 Suppl 2:S159–S170.

19. Rice TW, Wheeler AP, Thompson BT, deBoisblanc BP, et al. Enteral omega-3 fatty acid, gamma-linolenic acid, and antioxidant supplementation in acute lung injury. *JAMA: The Journal of the American Medical Association* 2011;306:1574–1581.

20. Carroll KK. Dietary proteins and amino acids—Their effects on cholesterol metabolism. In: Gibney MJ and Kritchevsky D, eds. *Current topics in nutrition and disease, volume 8: Animal and vegetable protein in lipid metabolism and atherosclerosis.* New York: Alan R. Liss, 1983.

21. Guallar E, Sanz-Gallardo MI, van't Veer P, Bode P, et al. Mercury, fish oils, and the risk of myocardial infarction. *New England Journal of Medicine* 2002;347:1747–1754.

22. Salonen JT, Seppänen K, Nyyssönen K, Korpela H, et al. Intake of mercury from fish, lipid peroxidation, and the risk of myocardial infarction and coronary, cardiovascular, and any death in eastern Finnish men. *Circulation* 1995;91:645–655.

23. Mozaffarian D and Rimm EB. Fish intake, contaminants, and human health: Evaluating the risks and the benefits. *JAMA: The Journal of the American Medical Association* 2006;296:1885–1899.

24. Abelsohn A, Vanderlinden LD, Scott F, Archbold JA, and Brown TL. Healthy fish consumption and reduced mercury exposure: Counseling women in their reproductive years. *Canadian Family Physician* 2011;57:26–30.

25. He K. Fish, long-chain omega-3 polyunsaturated fatty acids and prevention of cardiovascular disease—Eat fish or take fish oil supplement? *Progress in Cardiovascular Diseases* 2009;52:95–114.

26. Hooper L, Thompson RL, Harrison RA, Summerbell CD, et al. Risks and benefits of omega 3 fats for mortality, cardiovascular disease, and cancer: Systematic review. *BMJ* 2006;332:752–760.

27. Esselstyn CB Jr., Ellis SG, Medendorp SV, and Crowe TD. A strategy to arrest and reverse coronary artery disease: A 5-year longitudinal study of a single physician's practice. *Journal of Family Practice* 1995;41:560–568.

28. Willcox DC, Willcox BJ, Todoriki H, and Suzuki M. The Okinawan diet: Health implications of a low-calorie, nutrient-dense, antioxidant-rich dietary pattern low in glycemic load. *Journal of the American College of Nutrition* 2009;28 Suppl:500S–516S.

29. Sanders TA. DHA status of vegetarians. *Prostaglandins, Leukotrienes, and Essential Fatty Acids* 2009;81:137–141.

CHAPTER 8

1. Applied Research Program, National Cancer Institute. Usual intake of total grains, 2001–2004. April 2, 2014. http://riskfactor.cancer.gov/diet/usualintakes/pop/grains_all.html.

2. Krebs-Smith SM, Guenther PM, Subar AF, Kirkpatrick SI, and Dodd KW. Americans do not meet federal dietary recommendations. *Journal of Nutrition* 2010;140:1832–1838.

3. Applied Research Program, National Cancer Institute. Usual intake of whole grains, 2001–2004. April 2, 2014. http://riskfactor.cancer.gov/diet/usualintakes/pop/grains_whl.html.

4. Bachman JL, Reedy J, Subar AF, and Krebs-Smith SM. Sources of food group intakes among the US population, 2001-2002. *Journal of the American Dietetic Association* 2008;108:804–814.

5. Davis W. *Wheat belly: Lose the wheat, lose the weight, and find your path back to health.* Emmaus, PA: Rodale, 2011.

6. Sapone A, Bai JC, Ciacci C, Dolinsek J., et al. Spectrum of gluten-related disorders: Consensus on new nomenclature and classification. *BMC Medicine* 2012;10:13.

7. Boyce JA, Assa'ad A, Burks AW, Jones SM, et al. *Guidelines for the diagnosis and management of food allergy in the United States: Report of the NIAID-sponsored expert panel.* NIH Publication No. 11-7700. Bethesda, MD: National Institutes of Health, December 2010. http://www.niaid.nih.gov/topics/foodallergy/clinical/documents/faguidelinesexecsummary.pdf.

8. Rona RJ, Keil T, Summers C, Gislason D, et al. The prevalence of food allergy: A meta-analysis. *Journal of Allergy and Clinical Immunology* 2007;120:638–646.

9. Zuidmeer L, Goldhahn K, Rona RJ, Gislason D, et al. The prevalence of plant food allergies: A systematic review. *Journal of Allergy and Clinical Immunology* 2008;121:1210–1218.e4.

10. Rashtak S and Murray JA. Celiac disease in the elderly. *Gastroenterology Clinics of North America* 2009;38:433–446.

11. Fasano A, Berti I, Gerarduzzi T, Not T, et al. Prevalence of celiac disease in at-risk and not-at-risk groups in the United States: A large multicenter study. *Archives of Internal Medicine* 2003;163:286–292.

12. Fasano A and Catassi C. Celiac disease. *New England Journal of Medicine* 2012;367:2419–2426.

13. Kellogg EA. Evolutionary history of the grasses. *Plant Physiology* 2001;125:1198–1205.

14. Karell K, Louka AS, Moodie SJ, Ascher H, et al. HLA types in celiac disease patients not carrying the DQA1*05-DQB1*02 (DQ2) heterodimer: Results from the European Genetics Cluster on Celiac Disease. *Human Immunology* 2003;64:469–477.

15. Trynka G, Wijmenga C, and van Heel DA. A genetic perspective on coeliac disease. *Trends in Molecular Medicine* 2010;16:537–550.

16. Farrell RJ and Kelly CP. Celiac disease and refractory celiac disease. In: Sleisenger MH, Feldman M, Friedman LS, and Brandt LJ, eds. *Sleisenger and Fordtran's gastrointestinal and liver disease: Pathophysiology, diagnosis, management.* 9th ed. Philadelphia: Saunders/Elsevier, 2010.

17. Simell S, Hoppu S, Hekkala A, Ståhlberg MR, et al. Fate of five celiac disease-associated antibodies during normal diet in genetically at-risk children observed from birth in a natural history study. *American Journal of Gastroenterology* 2007;102:2026–2035.

18. Matysiak-Budnik T, Malamut G, de Serre NP-M, Grosdidier E, et al. Long-term follow-up of 61 coeliac patients diagnosed in childhood: Evolution toward latency is possible on a normal diet. *Gut* 2007;56:1379–1386.

19. Myléus A, Hernell O, Gothefors L, Hammarström ML, et al. Early infections are associated with increased risk for celiac disease: An incident case-referent study. *BMC Pediatrics* 2012;12:194.

20. Fasano A and Catassi C. Early feeding practices and their impact on development of celiac disease. *Nestlé Nutrition Workshop Series: Pediatric Programme* 2011;68:201–209.

21. Shamir R. Can feeding practices during infancy change the risk for celiac disease? *Israel Medical Association Journal: IMAJ* 2012;14:50–52.

22. DePaolo RW, Abadie V, Tang F, Fehlner-Peach H, et al. Co-adjuvant effects of retinoic acid and IL-15 induce inflammatory immunity to dietary antigens. *Nature* 2011;471:220–224.

23. Brown K, DeCoffe D, Molcan E, and Gibson DL. Diet-induced dysbiosis of the intestinal microbiota and the effects on immunity and disease. *Nutrients* 2012;4:1095–1119.

CHAPTER 9

1. Salmi TT, Hervonen K, Kautiainen H, Collin P, and Reunala T. Prevalence and incidence of dermatitis herpetiformis: A 40-year prospective study from Finland. *British Journal of Dermatology* 2011;165:354–359.

2. Sapone A, Bai JC, Ciacci C, Dolinsek J, et al. Spectrum of gluten-related disorders: Consensus on new nomenclature and classification. *BMC Medicine* 2012;10:13.

3. Toscano V, Conti FG, Anastasi E, Mariani P, et al. Importance of gluten in the induction of endocrine autoantibodies and organ dysfunction in adolescent celiac patients. *American Journal of Gastroenterology* 2000;95:1742–1748.

4. Mahmud FH, Murray JA, Kudva YC, Zinsmeister AR, et al. Celiac disease in type 1 diabetes mellitus in a North American community: Prevalence, serologic screening, and clinical features. *Mayo Clinic Proceedings* 2005;80:1429–1434.

5. Funda DP, Kaas A, Bock T, Tlaskalova-Hogenova H, and Buschard K. Gluten-free diet prevents diabetes in NOD mice. *Diabetes/Metabolism Research and Reviews* 1999;15:323–327.

6. Pastore MR, Bazzigaluppi E, Belloni C, Arcovio C, et al. Six months of gluten-free diet do not influence autoantibody titers, but improve insulin secretion in subjects at high risk for type 1 diabetes. *Journal of Clinical Endocrinology and Metabolism* 2003;88:162–165.

7. Elliott RB, Reddy SN, Bibby NJ, and Kida K. Dietary prevention of diabetes in the non-obese diabetic mouse. *Diabetologia* 1988;31:62–64.

8. van Belle TL, Coppieters KT, and von Herrath MG. Type 1 diabetes: Etiology, immunology, and therapeutic strategies. *Physiological Reviews* 2011;91:79–118.

9. Knip M, Virtanen SM, Seppä K, Ilonen J, et al. Dietary intervention in infancy and later signs of beta-cell autoimmunity. *New England Journal of Medicine* 2010;363:1900–1908.

10. Martinez SW. *Introduction of new food products with voluntary health- and nutrition-related claims, 1989-2010.* Economic Information Bulletin No. 108. Washington, DC: US Department of Agriculture, Economic Research Service, February 2013. www.ers.usda.gov/media/1037958/eib108.pdf

11. Carroccio A, Mansueto P, Iacono G, Soresi M, et al. Non-celiac wheat sensitivity diagnosed by double-blind placebo-controlled challenge: Exploring a new clinical entity. *American Journal of Gastroenterology* 2012;107:1898–1906.

12. Biesiekierski JR, Newnham ED, Irving PM, Barrett JS, et al. Gluten causes gastrointestinal symptoms in subjects without celiac disease: A double-blind

randomized placebo-controlled trial. *American Journal of Gastroenterology* 2011;106:508–514.

13. Lundin KE and Alaedini A. Non-celiac gluten sensitivity. *Gastrointestinal Endoscopy Clinics of North America* 2012;22:723–734.

14. Sverker A, Hensing G, and Hallert C. "Controlled by food"—Lived experiences of coeliac disease. *Journal of Human Nutrition and Dietetics* 2005;18:171–180.

CHAPTER 10

1. Riddle J and McEvoy M. What are the basic requirements for organic certification? Washington State Department of Agriculture, December 20, 2006. http://agr.wa.gov/foodanimal/organic/Certificate/2006/OrganicRequirementsSimplified.pdf.

2. Heaton S. *Organic farming, food quality and human health.* Bristol, UK: Soil Association, 2001.

3. Magkos F, Arvaniti F, and Zampelas A. Organic food: Buying more safety or just peace of mind? A critical review of the literature. *Critical Reviews in Food Science and Nutrition* 2006;46:23–56.

4. Worthington V. Nutritional quality of organic versus conventional fruits, vegetables, and grains. *Journal of Alternative and Complementary Medicine* 2001;7:161–173.

5. Magkos F, Arvaniti F, and Zampelas A. Organic food: Nutritious food or food for thought? A review of the evidence. *International Journal of Food Sciences and Nutrition* 2003;54:357–371.

6. Benbrook C, Zhao X, Yanez J, Davies N, and Andrews P. *New evidence confirms the nutritional superiority of plant-based organic foods.* Washington, DC: Organic Center, 2008.

7. Dangour AD, Dodhia SK, Hayter A, Allen E, et al. Nutritional quality of organic foods: A systematic review. *American Journal of Clinical Nutrition* 2009;90:680–685.

8. Smith-Spangler C, Brandeau ML, Hunter GE, Bavinger JC, et al. Are organic foods safer or healthier than conventional alternatives? A systematic review. *Annals of Internal Medicine* 2012;157:348–366.

9. Daley CA, Abbott A, Doyle PS, Nader GA, and Larson S. A review of fatty acid profiles and antioxidant content in grass-fed and grain-fed beef. *Nutrition Journal* 2010;9:10.

10. Baker BP, Benbrook CM, Groth E 3rd, and Lutz Benbrook K. Pesticide residues in conventional, integrated pest management (IPM)-grown and organic foods: Insights from three US data sets. *Food Additives and Contaminants* 2002;19:427–446.

11. Lu C, Barr DB, Pearson MA, and Waller LA. Dietary intake and its contribution to longitudinal organophosphorus pesticide exposure in urban/suburban children. *Environmental Health Perspectives* 2008;116:537–542.

12. Lu C, Toepel K, Irish R, Fenske RA, et al. Organic diets significantly lower children's dietary exposure to organophosphorus pesticides. *Environmental Health Perspectives* 2006;114:260–263.

13. Calvert GM, Karnik J, Mehler L, Beckman J, et al. Acute pesticide poisoning among agricultural workers in the United States, 1998-2005. *American Journal of Industrial Medicine* 2008;51:883–898.

14. Blair A and Freeman LB. Epidemiologic studies in agricultural populations: Observations and future directions. *Journal of Agromedicine* 2009;14:125–131.

15. Infante-Rivard C and Weichenthal S. Pesticides and childhood cancer: An update of Zahm and Ward's 1998 review. *Journal of Toxicology and Environmental Health: Part B, Critical Reviews* 2007;10:81–99.

16. Vinson F, Merhi M, Baldi I, Raynal H, and Gamet-Payrastre L. Exposure to pesticides and risk of childhood cancer: A meta-analysis of recent epidemiological studies. *Occupational and Environmental Medicine* 2011;68:694–702.

17. American Academy of Pediatrics. Policy statement: Pesticide exposure in children. *Pediatrics* 2012;130:e1757–e1763.

18. Dangour AD, Lock K, Hayter A, Aikenhead A, et al. Nutrition-related health effects of organic foods: A systematic review. *American Journal of Clinical Nutrition* 2010;92:203–210.

19. Campbell TC and Campbell TM. *The China Study: The most comprehensive study of nutrition ever conducted and the startling implications for diet, weight loss, and long-term health.* Dallas: BenBella Books, 2005.

20. Youngman LD and Campbell TC. The sustained development of preneoplastic lesions depends on high protein intake. *Nutrition and Cancer* 1992;18:131–142.

21. Crinnion WJ. Polychlorinated biphenyls: Persistent pollutants with immunological, neurological, and endocrinological consequences. *Alternative Medicine Reviews* 2011;16:5-13.

22. Jaga K and Duvvi H. Risk reduction for DDT toxicity and carcinogenesis through dietary modification. *Journal of the Royal Society for the Promotion of Health* 2001;121:107–113.

23. Environmental Working Group. EWG's 2014 shopper's guide to pesticides in produce. April 2014. www.ewg.org/foodnews.

24. Fernandez-Cornejo J, Wechsler S, Livingston M, and Mitchell L. *Genetically engineered crops in the United States.* Economic Research Report No. 162. Washington, DC: US Department of Agriculture, 2014.

25. Benbrook C. Impacts of genetically engineered crops on pesticide use in the U.S.—The first sixteen years. *Environmental Sciences Europe* 2012;24:1–13.

26. Owen M. Herbicide-resistant weeds in genetically engineered crops: Statement before the Subcommittee on Domestic Policy, Committee on Oversight and Government Reform, US House of Representatives, July 28, 2010.

27. Domingo JL and Gine Bordonaba J. A literature review on the safety assessment of genetically modified plants. *Environment International* 2011;37:734–742.

28. Seralini GE, Cellier D, and de Vendomois JS. New analysis of a rat feeding study with a genetically modified maize reveals signs of hepatorenal toxicity. *Archives of Environmental Contamination and Toxicology* 2007;52:596–602.

29. deVenomois JS, Roullier F, Cellier D, and Seralini GE. A comparison of the effects of three GM corn varieties on mammalian health. *International Journal of Biological Sciences* 2009;5:706–726.

30. Snell C, Bernheim A, Berge JB, Kuntz M, et al. Assessment of the health impact of GM plant diets in long-term and multigenerational animal feeding trials: A literature review. *Food and Chemical Toxicology* 2012;50:1134–1148.

31. Seralini GE, Clair E, Mesnage R, Gress S, et al. Long term toxicity of a Roundup herbicide and a Roundup-tolerant genetically modified maize. *Food and Chemical Toxicology* 2012;50:4221–4231.

32. Seralini GE, Mesnage R, Defarge N, Gress S, et al. Answers to critics: Why there is a long term toxicity due to a Roundup-tolerant genetically modified maize and to a Roundup herbicide. *Food and Chemical Toxicology* 2013;53:476–483.

33. Editors. Do Seed Companies Control GM Crop Research? *Scientific American,* July 20, 2009. www.scientificamerican.com/article.cfm?id=do-seed-companies-control-gm-crop-research. [editorial]

34. Robinson C and Latham J. The Goodman affair: Monsanto targets the heart of science. Independent Science News, May 20, 2013. www.independentsciencenews.org/science-media/the-goodman-affair-monsanto-targets-the-heart-of-science.

35. Thomson Reuters. National Survey of Healthcare Consumers: Genetically engineered food. October, 2010. www.justlabelit.org/wp-content/uploads/2011/09/NPR_report_GeneticEngineeredFood-1.pdf.

CHAPTER 11

1. Bailey RL, Gahche JJ, Miller PE, Thomas PR, and Dwyer JT. Why US adults use dietary supplements. *JAMA Internal Medicine* 2013;173:355–361.

2. Marik PE and Varon J. Omega-3 dietary supplements and the risk of cardiovascular events: A systematic review. *Clinical Cardiology* 2009;32:365–372.

3. Kwak SM, Myung SK, Lee YJ, and Seo HG. Efficacy of omega-3 fatty acid supplements (eicosapentaenoic acid and docosahexaenoic acid) in the secondary prevention of cardiovascular disease: A meta-analysis of randomized, double-blind, placebo-controlled trials. *Archives of Internal Medicine* 2012;172:686–694.

4. Rizos EC, Ntzani EE, Bika E, Kostapanos MS, and Elisaf MS. Association between omega-3 fatty acid supplementation and risk of major cardiovascular disease events: A systematic review and meta-analysis. *JAMA: The Journal of the American Medical Association* 2012;308:1024–1033.

5. Munro IA and Garg ML. Dietary supplementation with long chain omega-3 polyunsaturated fatty acids and weight loss in obese adults. *Obesity Research and Clinical Practice* 2013;7:e173–e181.

6. Mozurkewich EL, Clinton CM, Chilimigras JL, Hamilton SE, et al. The Mothers, Omega-3, and Mental Health Study: A double-blind, randomized controlled trial. *American Journal of Obstetrics and Gynecology* 2013;208:313.e1–313.e9.

7. Barbadoro P, Annino I, Ponzio E, Romanelli RM, et al. Fish oil supplementation reduces cortisol basal levels and perceived stress: A randomized, placebo-controlled trial in abstinent alcoholics. *Molecular Nutrition and Food Research* 2013;57:1110–1114.

8. Sydenham E, Dangour AD, and Lim WS. Omega 3 fatty acid for the prevention of cognitive decline and dementia. *Cochrane Database of Systematic Reviews* 2012;6:CD005379.

9. Harris WS. n-3 Fatty acids and serum lipoproteins: Human studies. *American Journal of Clinical Nutrition* 1997;65:1645S–1654S.

10. Harris WS, Ginsberg HN, Arunakul N, Shachter NS, et al. Safety and efficacy of Omacor in severe hypertriglyceridemia. *Journal of Cardiovascular Risk* 1997;4:385–391.

11. Pownall HJ, Brauchi D, Kilinc C, Osmundsen K, et al. Correlation of serum triglyceride and its reduction by omega-3 fatty acids with lipid transfer activity and the neutral lipid compositions of high-density and low-density lipoproteins. *Atherosclerosis* 1999;143:285–297.

12. Lee MW, Park JK, Hong JW, Kim KJ, et al. Beneficial effects of omega-3 fatty acids on low density lipoprotein particle size in patients with type 2 diabetes already under statin therapy. *Diabetes and Metabolism Journal* 2013;37:207–211.

13. Rosenson R. Approach to the patient with hypertriglyceridemia. UpToDate.com, January 24, 2014. www.uptodate.com/contents/approach-to-the-patient-with-hypertriglyceridemia.

14. Ginsberg HN, Elam MB, Lovato LC, Crouse JR 3rd, et al. Effects of combination lipid therapy in type 2 diabetes mellitus. *New England Journal of Medicine* 2010;362:1563–1574.

15. Mozaffarian D, Lemaitre RN, King IB, Song X, et al. Plasma phospholipid long-chain omega-3 fatty acids and total and cause-specific mortality in older adults: A cohort study. *Annals of Internal Medicine* 2013;158:515–525.

16. Esselstyn CB Jr., Ellis SG, Medendorp SV, and Crowe TD. A strategy to arrest and reverse coronary artery disease: A 5-year longitudinal study of a single physician's practice. *Journal of Family Practice* 1995;41:560–568.

17. National Institutes of Health State-of-the-Science Panel. National Institutes of Health State-of-the-Science Conference Statement: Multivitamin/mineral supplements and chronic disease prevention. *American Journal of Clinical Nutrition* 2007;85:257S–264S.

18. Honarbakhsh S and Schachter M. Vitamins and cardiovascular disease. *British Journal of Nutrition* 2009;101:1113–1131.

19. Office of Dietary Supplements, National Institutes of Health. Multivitamin/mineral supplements: Fact sheet for health professionals. January 7, 2013. http://ods.od.nih.gov/pdf/factsheets/MVMS-HealthProfessional.pdf.

20. Albanes D, Heinonen OP, Huttunen JK, Taylor PR, et al. Effects of alpha-tocopherol and beta-carotene supplements on cancer incidence in the Alpha-Tocopherol Beta-Carotene Cancer Prevention Study. *American Journal of Clinical Nutrition* 1995;62:1427S–1430S.

21. Age-Related Eye Disease Study Research Group. A randomized, placebo-controlled, clinical trial of high-dose supplementation with vitamins C and E, beta carotene, and zinc for age-related macular degeneration and vision loss: AREDS report no. 8. *Archives of Ophthalmology* 2001;119:1417–1436.

22. Chew EY, Clemons TE, Agron E, Sperduto RD, et al. Long-term effects of vitamins C and E, beta-carotene, and zinc on age-related macular degeneration: AREDS report no. 35. *Ophthalmology* 2013;120:1604-11.e4.

23. Age-Related Eye Disease Study Research Group. A randomized, placebo-controlled, clinical trial of high-dose supplementation with vitamins C and E and beta carotene for age-related cataract and vision loss: AREDS report no. 9. *Archives of Ophthalmology* 2001;119:1439–1452.

24. Bronstein AC, Spyker DA, Cantilena LR Jr, Green JL, et al. 2008 Annual report of the American Association of Poison Control Centers' National Poison Data System (NPDS): 26th annual report. *Clinical Toxicology (Philadelphia)* 2009;47:911–1084.

25. Institute of Medicine. *Dietary reference intakes for vitamin A, vitamin K, arsenic, boron, chromium, copper, iodine, iron, manganese, molybdenum, nickel, silicon, vanadium, and zinc.* Washington, DC: National Academies Press, 2001.

26. Uusi-Rasi K, Karkkainen MU, and Lamberg-Allardt CJ. Calcium intake in health maintenance—A systematic review. *Food and Nutrition Research* 2013;57:21082.

27. Institute of Medicine. *Dietary Reference Intakes for Calcium and Vitamin D.* Washington, DC: National Academies Press, 2011.

28. Moyer VA. Vitamin D and calcium supplementation to prevent fractures in adults: U.S. Preventive Services Task Force recommendation statement. *Annals of Internal Medicine* 2013;158:691–696.

29. Bolland MJ, Avenell A, Baron JA, Grey A, et al. Effect of calcium supplements on risk of myocardial infarction and cardiovascular events: Meta-analysis. *BMJ* 2010;341:c3691.

30. Appleby P, Roddam A, Allen N, and Key T. Comparative fracture risk in vegetarians and nonvegetarians in EPIC-Oxford. *European Journal of Clinical Nutrition* 2007;61:1400–1406.

31. Sellmeyer DE, Stone KL, Sebastian A, and Cummings SR. A high ratio of dietary animal to vegetable protein increases the rate of bone loss and the risk of fracture in postmenopausal women. Study of Osteoporotic Fractures Research Group. *American Journal of Clinical Nutrition* 2001;73:118–122.

32. Howe TE, Shea B, Dawson LJ, Downie F, et al. Exercise for preventing and treating osteoporosis in postmenopausal women. *Cochrane Database of Systematic Reviews* 2011:CD000333.

33. Office of Dietary Supplements, National Institutes of Health. Vitamin D: Fact sheet for health professionals. June 24, 2011. http://ods.od.nih.gov/pdf/factsheets/VitaminD-HealthProfessional.pdf.

34. Holick MF, Binkley NC, Bischoff-Ferrari HA, Gordon CM, et al. Guidelines for preventing and treating vitamin D deficiency and insufficiency revisited. *Journal of Clinical Endocrinology and Metabolism* 2012;97:1153–1158.

35. Holick MF. Vitamin D deficiency. *New England Journal of Medicine* 2007;357:266–281.

36. Misra M, Pacaud D, Petryk A, Collett-Solberg PF, and Kappy M. Vitamin D deficiency in children and its management: Review of current knowledge and recommendations. *Pediatrics* 2008;122:398–417.

37. Specker BL, Valanis B, Hertzberg V, Edwards N, and Tsang RC. Sunshine exposure and serum 25-hydroxyvitamin D concentrations in exclusively breast-fed infants. *Journal of Pediatrics* 1985;107:372–376.

38. Watanabe F, Yabuta Y, Tanioka Y, and Bito T. Biologically active vitamin B_{12} compounds in foods for preventing deficiency among vegetarians and elderly subjects. *Journal of Agricultural and Food Chemistry* 2013;61:6769–6775.

39. Stabler SP. Vitamin B_{12} deficiency. *New England Journal of Medicine* 2013;368:149–160.

40. De Rosa A, Rossi F, Lieto M, Bruno R, et al. Subacute combined degeneration of the spinal cord in a vegan. *Clinical Neurology and Neurosurgery* 2012;114:1000–1002.

41. Brocadello F, Levedianos G, Piccione F, Manara R, and Pesenti FF. Irreversible subacute sclerotic combined degeneration of the spinal cord in a vegan subject. *Nutrition* 2007;23:622–624.

42. Campbell M, Lofters WS, and Gibbs WN. Rastafarianism and the vegans syndrome. *British Medical Journal* 1982;285:1617–1618.

43. Kwok T, Lee J, Lam L, and Woo J. Vitamin B_{12} supplementation did not improve cognition but reduced delirium in demented patients with vitamin B_{12} deficiency. *Archives of Gerontology and Geriatrics* 2008;46:273–282.

44. Oh R and Brown DL. Vitamin B_{12} deficiency. *American Family Physician* 2003;67:979–986.

45. Lindenbaum J, Healton EB, Savage DG, Brust JC, et al. Neuropsychiatric disorders caused by cobalamin deficiency in the absence of anemia or macrocytosis. *New England Journal of Medicine* 1988;318:1720–1728.

46. Kwok T, Chook P, Qiao M, Tam L, et al. Vitamin B_{12} supplementation improves arterial function in vegetarians with subnormal vitamin B_{12} status. *Journal of Nutrition, Health and Aging* 2012;16:569–573.

47. Oner T, Guven B, Tavli V, Mese T, et al. Postural orthostatic tachycardia syndrome (POTS) and vitamin B_{12} deficiency in adolescents. *Pediatrics* 2014;133:e138–e142.

48. Lewerin C, Nilsson-Ehle H, Jacobsson S, Johansson H, et al. Low holotranscobalamin and cobalamins predict incident fractures in elderly men: The MrOS Sweden. *Osteoporosis International* 2014;25:131–140.

49. Dhonukshe-Rutten RA, van Dusseldorp M, Schneede J, de Groot LC, and van Staveren WA. Low bone mineral density and bone mineral content are associated with low cobalamin status in adolescents. *European Journal of Nutrition* 2005;44:341–347.

50. Yang HT, Lee M, Hong KS, Ovbiagele B, and Saver JL. Efficacy of folic acid supplementation in cardiovascular disease prevention: An updated meta-analysis of randomized controlled trials. *European Journal of Internal Medicine* 2012;23:745–754.

51. Pepper MR and Black MM. B_{12} in fetal development. *Seminars in Cell and Developmental Biology* 2011;22:619–623.

52. Lam JR, Schneider JL, Zhao W, and Corley DA. Proton pump inhibitor and histamine 2 receptor antagonist use and vitamin B_{12} deficiency. *JAMA: The Journal of the American Medical Association* 2013;310:2435–2342.

53. Crane M and Sample C. Vitamin B_{12} studies in total vegetarians (vegans). *Journal of Nutritional Medicine* 1994;4:12.

CHAPTER 12

1. Waterland RA and Jirtle RL. Transposable elements: Targets for early nutritional effects on epigenetic gene regulation. *Molecular and Cellular Biology* 2003;23:5293–5300.

2. Waterland RA, Travisano M, Tahiliani KG, Rached MT, and Mirza S. Methyl donor supplementation prevents transgenerational amplification of obesity. *International Journal of Obesity (London)* 2008;32:1373–1379.

3. Skogen JC and Overland S. The fetal origins of adult disease: A narrative review of the epidemiological literature. *JRSM Short Reports* 2012;3:59.

4. Gaillard R, Durmus B, Hofman A, Mackenbach JP, et al. Risk factors and outcomes of maternal obesity and excessive weight gain during pregnancy. *Obesity* 2013;21:1046–1055.

5. Rasmussen KM and Yaktine AL, eds. *Weight gain during pregnancy: Reexamining the guidelines*. Committee to Reexamine IOM Pregnancy Weight Guidelines. Washington, DC: National Academies Press, 2009.

6. Streuling I, Beyerlein A, Rosenfeld E, Schukat B, and von Kries R. Weight gain and dietary intake during pregnancy in industrialized countries—A systematic review of observational studies. *Journal of Perinatal Medicine* 2011;39:123–129.

7. Stuebe AM, Oken E, and Gillman MW. Associations of diet and physical activity during pregnancy with risk for excessive gestational weight gain. *American Journal of Obstetrics and Gynecology* 2009;201:58. e1–58.e8.

8. Qiu C, Zhang C, Gelaye B, Enquobahrie DA, et al. Gestational diabetes mellitus in relation to maternal dietary heme iron and nonheme iron intake. *Diabetes Care* 2011;34:1564–1569.

9. Qiu C, Frederick IO, Zhang C, Sorensen TK, et al. Risk of gestational diabetes mellitus in relation to maternal egg and cholesterol intake. *American Journal of Epidemiology* 2011;173:649–658.

10. Koebnick C, Leitzmann R, Garcia AL, Heins UA, et al. Long-term effect of a plant-based diet on magnesium status during pregnancy. *European Journal of Clinical Nutrition* 2005;59:219–225.

11. Craig WJ and Mangels AR. Position of the American Dietetic Association: Vegetarian diets. *Journal of the American Dietetic Association* 2009;109:1266–1282.

12. De-Regil LM, Fernandez-Gaxiola AC, Dowswell T, and Pena-Rosas JP. Effects and safety of periconceptional folate supplementation for preventing birth defects. *Cochrane Database of Systematic Reviews* 2010:CD007950.

13. Hoyo C, Murtha AP, Schildkraut JM, Forman MR, et al. Folic acid supplementation before and during pregnancy in the Newborn Epigenetics STudy (NEST). *BMC Public Health* 2011;11:46.

14. Vollset SE, Clarke R, Lewington S, Ebbing M, et al. Effects of folic acid supplementation on overall and site-specific cancer incidence during the randomised trials: Meta-analyses of data on 50,000 individuals. *Lancet* 2013;381:1029–1036.

15. Yang HT, Lee M, Hong KS, Ovbiagele B, and Saver JL. Efficacy of folic acid supplementation in cardiovascular disease prevention: An updated meta-analysis of randomized controlled trials. *European Journal of Internal Medicine* 2012;23:745–754.

16. Agricultural Research Service, US Department of Agriculture. USDA National Nutrient Database for Standard Reference, Release 26.

17. Innis SM. Dietary omega 3 fatty acids and the developing brain. *Brain Research* 2008;1237:35-43.

18. Novak EM, Dyer RA, and Innis SM. High dietary omega-6 fatty acids contribute to reduced docosahexaenoic acid in the developing brain and inhibit secondary neurite growth. *Brain Research* 2008;1237:136–145.

19. Schulzke SM, Patole SK, and Simmer K. Long-chain polyunsaturated fatty acid supplementation in preterm infants. *Cochrane Database of Systematic Reviews* 2011:CD000375.

20. Simmer K, Patole SK, and Rao SC. Long-chain polyunsaturated fatty acid supplementation in infants born at term. *Cochrane Database of Systemic Reviews* 2011:CD000376.

21. Lawrence RM and Lawrence RA. Breastfeeding: More than just good nutrition. *Pediatrics in Review* 2011;32:267–280.

22. Klement E, Cohen RV, Boxman J, Joseph A, and Reif S. Breastfeeding and risk of inflammatory bowel disease: A systematic review with meta-analysis. *American Journal of Clinical Nutrition* 2004;80:1342–1352.

23. Breastfeeding and the use of human milk. *Pediatrics* 2012;129:e827–e841.

24. Beauchamp GK and Mennella JA. Flavor perception in human infants: Development and functional significance. *Digestion* 2011;83 Suppl 1:1–6.

25. Dettwyler KA. When to wean: Biological versus cultural perspectives. *Clinical Obstetrics and Gynecology* 2004;47:712–723.

26. Standing Committee on the Scientific Evaluation of Dietary Reference Intakes, Institute of Medicine. Institute of Medicine. *Dietary reference intakes for thiamin, riboflavin, niacin, vitamin B$_6$, folate, vitamin B$_{12}$, pantothenic acid, biotin, and choline.* Washington, DC: National Academy Press, 1998.

27. Wansink B. Nutritional gatekeepers and the 72% solution. *Journal of the American Dietetic Association* 2006;106:1324–1327.

CHAPTER 13

1. Norcross JC, Krebs PM, and Prochaska JO. Stages of change. *Journal of Clinical Psychology* 2011;67:143–154.

2. Whitlock EP, Orleans CT, Pender N, and Allan J. Evaluating primary care behavioral counseling interventions: An evidence-based approach. *American Journal of Preventive Medicine* 2002;22:267–284.

3. Wansink B. Convenient, attractive, and normative: The CAN approach to making children slim by design. *Childhood Obesity* 2013;9:277–278.

4. Painter JE, Wansink B, and Hieggelke JB. How visibility and convenience influence candy consumption. *Appetite* 2002;38:237–238.

5. Wansink B. From mindless eating to mindlessly eating better. *Physiology and Behavior* 2010;100:454–463.

6. Thomas JG, Bond DS, Phelan S, Hill JO, and Wing RR. Weight-loss maintenance for 10 years in the National Weight Control Registry. *American Journal of Preventive Medicine* 2014;46:17–23.

CHAPTER 14

1. Tal A and Wansink B. Fattening fasting: Hungry grocery shoppers buy more calories, not more food. *JAMA Internal Medicine* 2013;173:1146–1148.
2. Whole Grains Council. Whole grains A to Z. n.d. http://wholegrainscouncil.org/whole-grains-101/whole-grains-a-to-z.
3. Panel on Dietary Reference Intakes for Electrolytes and Water, Institute of Medicine. *Dietary Reference Intakes for water, potassium, sodium, chloride, and sulfate.* Washington, DC: National Academies Press, 2005.

CHAPTER 16

1. Lowe MR, Doshi SD, Katterman SN, and Feig EH. Dieting and restrained eating as prospective predictors of weight gain. *Frontiers in Psychology* 2013;4:577.
2. Mattes RD. Fat preference and adherence to a reduced-fat diet. *American Journal of Clinical Nutrition* 1993;57:373–381.
3. Bertino M, Beauchamp GK, and Engelman K. Long-term reduction in dietary sodium alters the taste of salt. *American Journal of Clinical Nutrition* 1982;36:1134–1144.
4. Avena NM, Rada P, and Hoebel BG. Sugar and fat bingeing have notable differences in addictive-like behavior. *Journal of Nutrition* 2009;139:623–628.
5. Baumeister RF and Tierney J. *Willpower: Rediscovering the greatest human strength.* New York: Penguin, 2011.
6. Vohs KD and Heatherton TF. Self-regulatory failure: A resource-depletion approach. *Psychological Science* 2000;11:249–254.
7. Vohs KD, Redden JP, and Rahinel R. Physical order produces healthy choices, generosity, and conventionality, whereas disorder produces creativity. *Psychological Science* 2013;24:1860–1867.
8. Wansink B, Shimizu M, and Brumberg A. How vegetables make the meal: Their hedonic and heroic impact on perceptions of the meal and of the preparer. *Public Health Nutrition* 2013;16:1988–1994.
9. Christakis NA and Fowler JH. The spread of obesity in a large social network over 32 years. *New England Journal of Medicine* 2007;357:370–379.
10. Christakis NA and Fowler JH. Social contagion theory: Examining dynamic social networks and human behavior. *Statistics in Medicine* 2013;32:556–577.
11. Whitlock EP, Orleans CT, Pender N, and Allan J. Evaluating primary care behavioral counseling interventions: An evidence-based approach. *American Journal of Preventive Medicine* 2002;22:267–284.

ACKNOWLEDGMENTS

I would like to acknowledge my wife, Erin Campbell, for making this book possible. She gave a great deal of her time and energy into making the book practical and reviewing and writing its recipes while finishing her residency, which was certainly no easy task. In addition, this book would not have been possible without the bottomless support provided by my parents, T. Colin and Karen Campbell. They have been my best teachers. My dad has provided invaluable professional and scientific mentorship for the past 15 years.

Beyond these personal supports, I have to thank Celeste Fine, my agent, and all the folks at Rodale. I am thrilled that Mary Ann Naples and the team believed in this project. I particularly want to acknowledge Jennifer Levesque for her editing and guidance and Christopher DeMarchis for his near daily efforts to keep me on track. Nancy Elgin truly improved my manuscript with her detailed editing work. There are many others, including Brent Gallenberger, Aly Mostel, and Susan Turner, who round out the team, some of whom I have not even met. Together we worked to create this book and to advance its success.

In addition, I want to acknowledge Eric Lindstrom and Jeremy Rose for help in marketing and web development. The team at the T. Colin Campbell Center for Nutrition Studies, including Jenny Miller, Anne Ledbetter, Sarah Dwyer, Juan Lube, and the rest of the staff are integral to the message in this book and my efforts to advance it.

I would also like to acknowledge the University of Rochester Medical Center, both the entire family medicine residency program and Betty Rabinowitz and the Primary Care Network, for allowing me the chance to pursue my passion for using nutrition and lifestyle in the prevention and treatment of illness.

And lastly, I would like to acknowledge my patients, who have been my best teachers when it comes to crafting a useful and engaging discussion about changing diet and lifestyle. Nothing about change is easy, particularly when it comes to food, but I have been inspired by the success some of you have had.

Underscored page references indicate boxed text and tables.

E

Eating out, 46–48, 186, 189
Eaton, S. Boyd, 18–19
Eczema, 85
Egg substitutions, 160
Eliminating problem foods, 38–41,
   146–47, 148
Enchiladas, 237
Environment, preparing for change,
   145–47, 148
Environmental exposures, genetic
   expression and, 127–28
Environmental toxins
   in fish, 75, 77–78, 78, 131
   pesticide residues, 105–8
Environmental Working Group, 107, 108
EPA (omega-3 fatty acid), 68, 72, 78,
   130–31
Epigenetics, 127–28, 131
Esselstyn, Ann, 168
Esselstyn, Caldwell, Jr., 6, 41
Essential fatty acids, 64–65, 65, 67.
   See also Omega-3 fatty acids;
   Omega-6 fatty acids
Estrogen, 56–58
Ethiopian restaurants, 48
Ethnic foods, 47–48, 159, 166
Ethnographic Atlas, 16
EWG's Shopper's Guide to Pesticides in
   Produce, 107, 108
Exercise, 191–92
Eye health, 118, 130–31

F

Family support. *See* Social support for
   diet changes
Farmers' markets, 101
Fast food, 47. *See also* Restaurants
Fasting, 19
Fatigue, 87
Fats, 59–70. *See also* Oils
   addiction to, 42–43
   cancer promotion of, 63–64
   fatty acids, 64–65, 65, 67
   in fish, 66–67, 72–74, 76
   in grass-fed vs. grain-fed meats, 103
   in plant foods, 28, 28, 162

preferences for, 181
   recommendations for, 164
   substitutions for, 160
Fatty acids, 64–65, 65, 67
Fiber, 29
Fish, 71–79
   cholesterol in, 74–75, 76
   genetically modified, 109
   mercury and, 75, 131
   omega-3 fatty acids and, 72–74, 76
   recommendations for, 77–78
   unsaturated fats in, 66–67
Fisher, Cathy, 168
Fish oil, 68. *See also* Fish
Flaxseed
   alpha-linolenic acid and, 78–79
   during pregnancy, 131
   how to use, 157
Folic acid, 129–30, 130
Food challenge tests for allergies,
   85–86
Food diaries, 149
Food industry, financial interests of,
   10–11
Fortified foods
   folate in, 129
   for children, 136
   minerals in, 30
   vitamin B_{12} in, 124
   vitamin D in, 120
French Toast, 207
Friends and family. *See* Social support
   for diet changes
Frozen foods, recommended, 157
Fruit
   Amazingly Delicious Date Fruit Pie,
      250
   Banana-Maple Oatmeal Cookies,
      246–47
   Berry Sauce, 205
   Best Banana Bread, 202
   Frozen Banana Cream, 246
   in sauces and dressings, 156
   Mango-Lime Bean Salad, 217
   Mixed Fruit Cobbler, 248
   Pineapple Sponge Cake, 245
   Pineapple Stir-Fry, 234
   Strawberry Vinaigrette, 216

G

Garlic, 156
Gender, sugar consumption and, 53–54
Genetically modified organisms
        (GMOs), 108–12
    animals, 109
    plants, 108–9
    safety of, 109–12
Genetic expression
    cancer and, 12
    celiac disease and, 87, 87, 88–89, 97–98
    epigenetics and, 127–28, 131
Gestational diabetes, 128–29
Ginger, 156
Gluten. *See* Wheat
Gluten ataxia, 86, 91–92
Gluten-free diets, 82–83, 93, 96–97
Gluten intolerance without celiac
        disease, 83–84, 92–96, 98
Glyphosate, 109
GMOs. *See* Genetically modified
        organisms
Goals for diet changes, 43–44. *See also*
        Success
Gorillas, heart disease in, 14–15
Grains. *See also* Wheat; Whole grains
    family tree of, 88
    refined vs. whole foods, 29, 30, 162–63
Grass-fed meats, 103–5, 104
Greek restaurants, 48
Greens
    alpha-linolenic acid and, 78–79
    calcium in, 120
    folate in, 129–30, 130
    Global Greens, 230–31
    organic vs. non-organic, 103–5, 104
    Rainbow Greens, 233
    Sautéed Baby Spinach, 230
    Sautéed Bok Choy, 230
    Steamed Kale, 229
Grocery stores, tips for, 159, 166
Gut bacteria, 12–13, 20

H

Habits, creating, 146–47, 181, 184
Heartburn medications, nutrient
        absorption and, 124

Heart disease
    calcium supplementation and, 120
    fish consumption and, 68, 72, 75–76
    in gorillas, 14–15
    low-carbohydrate diets and, 21–24
    meat and dairy consumption and, 6,
        12–13, 40–41
    mercury and, 75
    omega-3 fatty acids and, 73, 115–17
    resources for, 168
    treating, 6–7, 7, 41, 69–70
    unsaturated fats and, 68–69
    vitamin B_{12} and, 124
Hemoglobin, 80
Herbicides, 109
Histamine, 84
Home, preparing for change, 145–47
Hormones, soy foods and, 56–58
Human Milk Banking Association of
        North America, 133
Hummus, 156
    Traditional Low-Fat Hummus, 210–11
    Zucchini Pritti-Hummus Wrap, 210
Hunter-gatherer societies, 16, 18–19. *See
        also* Paleolithic diet
Hyperpalatable foods, 52–53

I

IBS, 94–95
Ice cream, 161
IgE (immunoglobulin E) antibodies, 84
Immunity
    allergies and, 84
    celiac disease and, 81, 86–90
Indian restaurants, 48
Infertility, 87
Inflammation
    allergic reactions and, 84–85
    celiac disease and, 81, 86–90
    foods for, 73–74, 102
Ingredient lists, 46–47. *See also* Labels,
        nutrition
Insecticides, 109–10
Institute of Medicine
    on bone health, 119
    on health weight during pregnancy, 128
    on vitamin D, 122

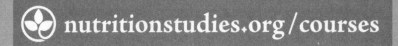